The Beginner's Guide
to
Joint Health

I0419605

Tips to Reduce the Pain
and
Keep Your Joints Healthy

RON KNESS

Published by:

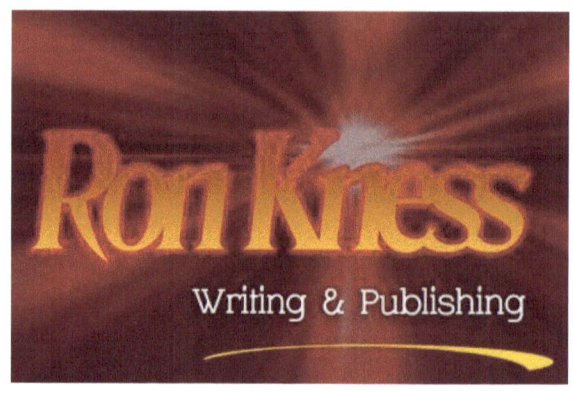

https://ronknesswriting.com

Ron Kness

Gold Canyon, AZ

United States of America

ISBN: 9781091040700

TABLE OF CONTENTS

INTRODUCTION

TO

JOINT HEALTH

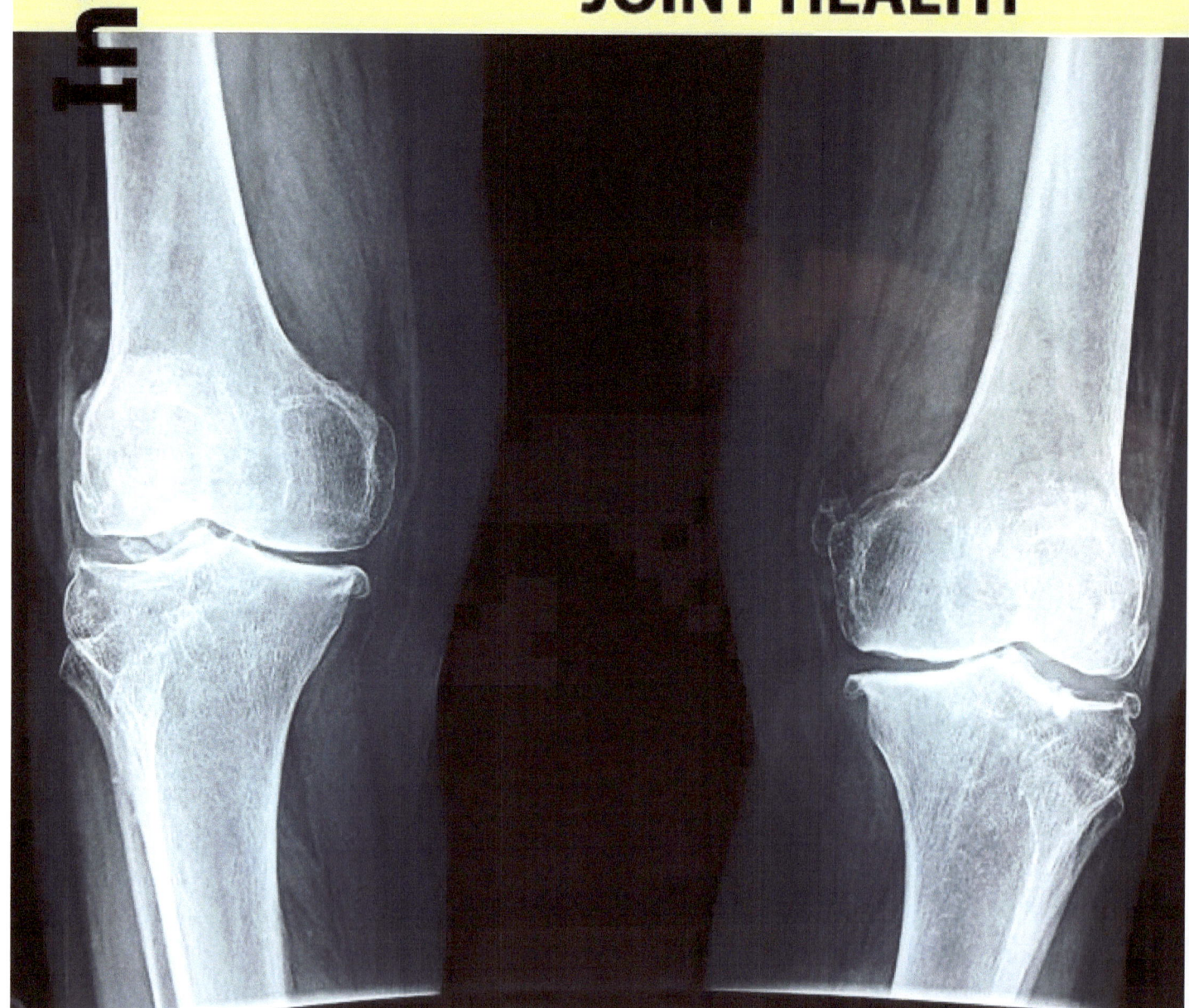

Introduction

If you've ever sat in awe watching children play, marvelling at the immense amount of energy and flexibility they have, you know that it's thanks to their healthy joints. But as you age, even bending down to pick something up from the floor can become an impossible feat.

So how do you deal with this?

While you can't really fight the process of aging, you can surely slow down the rate of damage inflicted on joints due to wear and tear. Learning how to nourish and take care of your joints will let you stay flexible for longer and yield relief for painful joints.

Let me share my story about joint pain with you. Joint health is a subject near and dear to my heart as I have osteoarthritis in my shoulders, wrists and hands. I was taking diclofenac prescribed by my doctor for the pain. And while it did help with the pain, unbeknownst to me it was interfering with the functioning of my kidneys. I didn't find that out until I went in for a hernia operation and the anesthesiologist mentioned that my kidney values were much higher than they should be for someone my age and in good shape.

He asked what medications I was taking and when I mentioned diclofenac, he said that was the one causing problems and that I should stop taking it and see if my doctor would prescribe something else. In the end, I stopped taking it and did not get a replacement. My kidney values were recently checked again a year later and have returned to normal. I can live with joint pain, but I can't live well without functioning kidneys.

What I have found now that works the best for me is exercise – one hour three times per week. And while I do have some pain on cold damp days, most days it is tolerable. This was a case where the side effects from the medication were worse than the condition it was treating.

Read on to see what it takes to keep yourself and your joints moving well as you age.

CHAPTER 1

WHY KEEP YOUR JOINTS HEALTHY

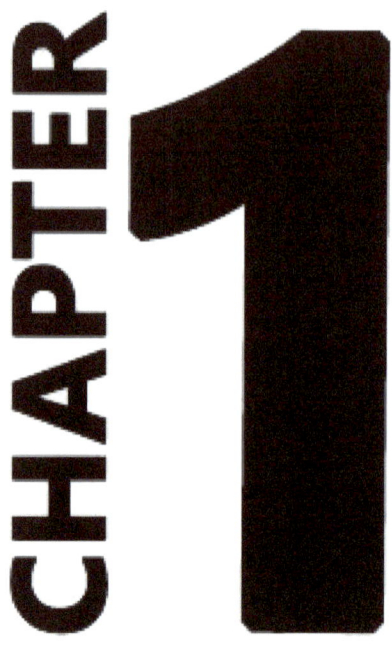

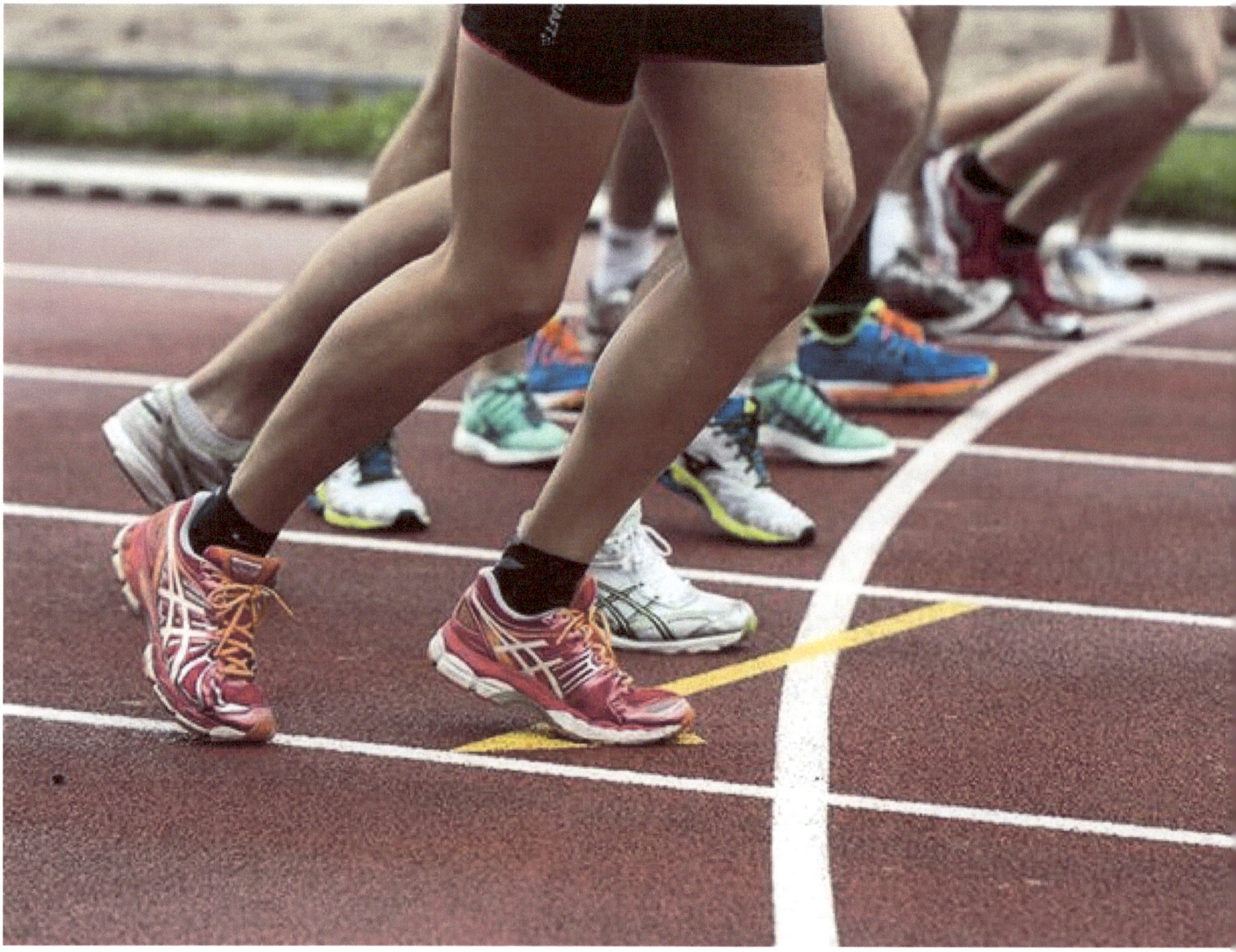

Chapter 1

Why Keep Your Joints Healthy?

Every time you sprint to catch the bus, score a point against your opposing team, or shoot pool with friends, you're using your extremely functional musculoskeletal system. This means a combination of bones, joints and muscles get you going where you want to go.

But muscles and bones don't work alone. Instead there are joints that link these together. While bones support your body's entire weight, your muscles pull your bones as you move. Joints are the connecting links that put both bones and muscles in motion.

Given the important functions of mobility and movement, it becomes crucial that you take good care of your joints. After all, you put them through so much wear and tear throughout your life.

Joints that aren't well taken care of become susceptible to injury, inflammation and general dislocation. As age catches up with you, you can feel the effects of overuse weathering away your joints. So keep your joints healthy at every stage of your life so they can keep you moving even in old age.

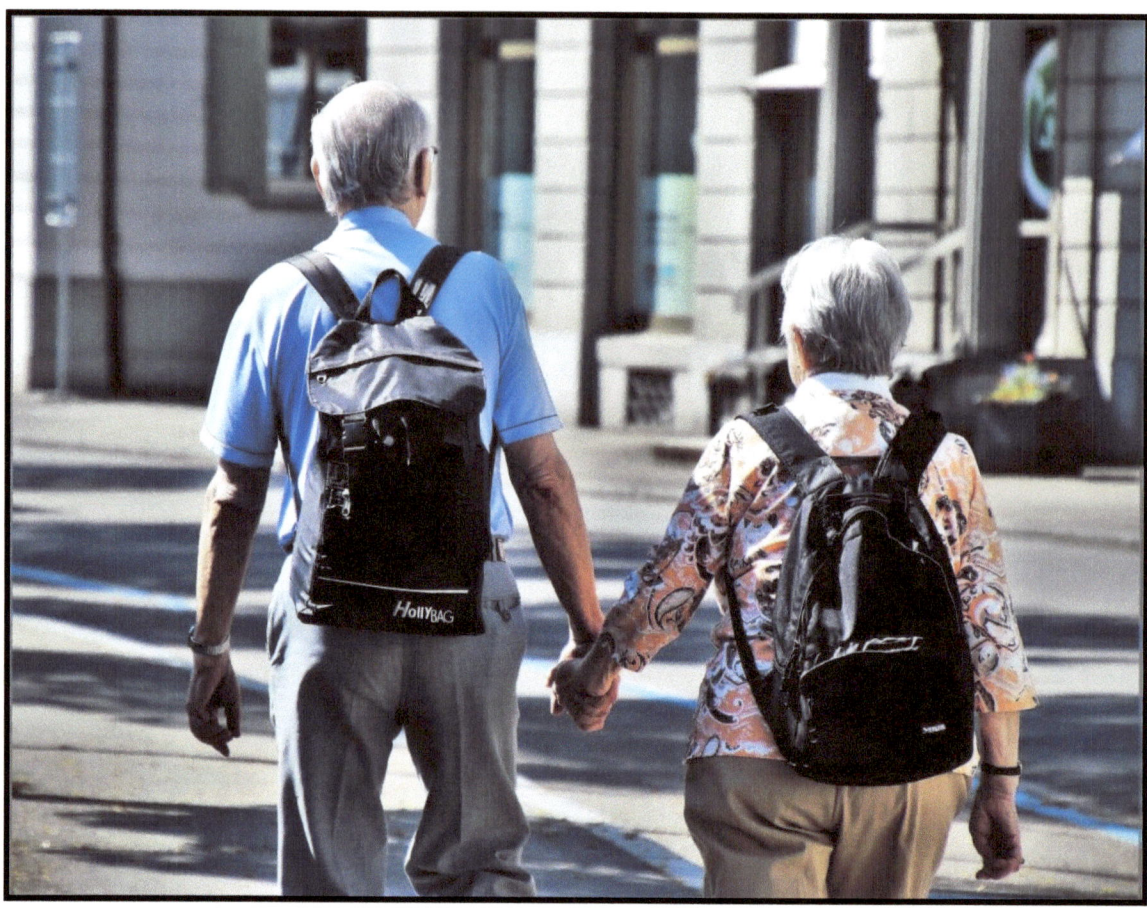

But before we look at ways to do so, here's a quick look at the anatomy of a joint so you can better understand what goes into keeping your joints healthy.

Which Bones Constitute a Joint?

Imagine if the skeleton had only one solid bone. That would make it very difficult to move. So instead nature solved this problem by dividing the skeleton into many bones, and creating joints where the bones intersect.

Joints are also known as articulations forming strong connections that join bones, teeth, and cartilage to one another. Now you have the freedom of movement in different ways and directions.

Some joints open and close like a hinge such as your knees and elbows, allowing you to straighten or bend your legs and arms. You sit down, stand up, pick up, and put down stuff using these joints without giving it a second thought.

Others joints are meant for more complicated movements such as your shoulder or hip joint. These allow for forward, backward, sideways, and rotating movements. Just think of everything you can do with these joints and you'll get an idea of how limited your movement can become if any of these joints suffer damage.

But not all joints are created equal. For instance, while joints like the knees provide stability, others like the wrist, ankles, and hips let you move, glide, skip, or run.

And just as their functions vary, so does their anatomy. Which means that you also need to take care of them in specific ways.

Some joints are purely made of tough collagen fiber while others have cartilage binding bones together. Yet others have something known as synovial fluid in between cartilage pads at the end of articulating bones.

So while you may think that all joints can be maintained using the same methods, you may need to rethink your joint-health strategy. Let's first take a look at the different types of joints found in the body before discussing how to take care of them.

Joints And How They Function

Each joint is specialized in its shape and structure to control the range of motion between the parts it connects.

For easier understanding, you may classify joints based on the function they perform or how much movement they allow. You can also do the same based on the structure of the joint, or the material that is present in the joint. This means looking at how the bones are attached to one another.

Both categories will let you divide joints into three broad classes:

- **Immovable or fixed joints.** These are typically fibrous joints that are held together by dense fibrous connective tissue. Think about the bony plates of the skull to get an idea. There are links or joints between the edges of these plates made of fibrous tissue. The point is to make them immovable to protect the brain.

- **Slightly movable or cartilaginous joints.** Here bones are held together by cartilage and allow for some degree of movement. An example could be the spine where each vertebra is linked by cartilage. With this arrangement, every vertebra moves in relation to the one above or below it, giving the spine its flexibility. This lets you bend forward, backward, or sideways without straining your back.

- **Freely movable or synovial joints.** This third type is the most abundantly found type in the body. Here, joints have a synovial cavity that contains a fluid. This synovial fluid lubricates the area and helps the joints move easily.

This type of joint allows the greatest range of movement letting you propel yourself in just about any direction. Examples include your elbows, knees, hips, and shoulders among others.

Synovial joints can further be divided into 6 types including the following:

- **Hinge** joints such as the fingers and toes
- **Ball and socket** joints such as the shoulders and hips
- **Pivot** joints such as the neck
- **Gliding** joints such as the wrist
- **Saddle** joints such as the thumb
- **Planar** joints such as the ankle

Healthy vs Painful Joints

Unlike many other health conditions, where it's not always possible to detect early warning signs of wear and tear, your joints are a different story. In fact, one of the first places where you feel your age is in your joints.

In most cases, joint issues generally develop over time and can make it hard for you to get around in everyday life. When things are going well, you won't feel any discomfort or pain, but if your joints start to give way, you may experience some of the symptoms discussed here.

The foremost among these is experiencing joint pain. This may mean you're exerting your joints too much or that you've already worn them out a fair bit.

If your joints become sore or tender to touch, it could indicate possible (internal) inflammation. Remember that inflammation isn't always visible to the eye and may continue for a while internally before symptoms become apparent externally.

Likewise, if you experience slow mobility and movement because your joints hurt, consider it another red flag. And if your joints offer little flexibility with a reduced range of motion, you may want to get a professional's opinion.

Another tell-tale sign of joint-health deterioration is creaking joints. If you hear clicking, creaking, or cracking sounds, or feel that your joints grate every time you move, you should become concerned about possible joint damage.

Plus, you should also be ware of your joint health if you happen to be overweight. Among other things, excessive weight is also associated with increased inflammation, a leading cause of joint discomfort.

If your work involves taxing your joints, such as lifting heavy objects, or even sitting for prolonged periods, you can start to develop joint issues as well. And finally, if you have family history of joint issues in the past, you may be more susceptible to developing certain joint-related conditions.

CHAPTER 2

COMMON JOINT PROBLEMS

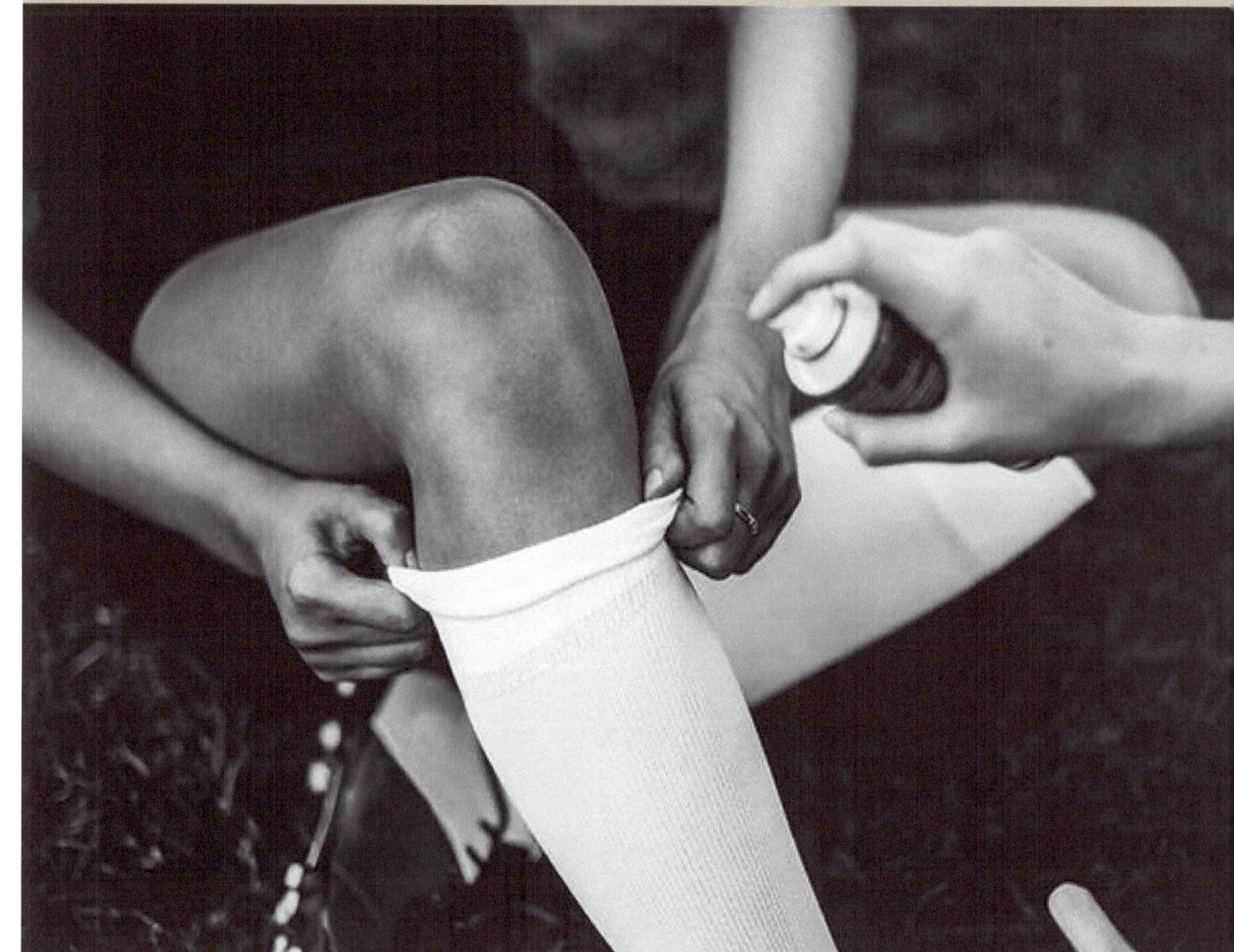

Chapter 2

Common Joint Problems

A common source of joint discomfort is inflammation. In fact, many of the problems associated with joint pain stem from inflammation. This can cause joints to become inflamed, swollen, stiff and even rickety when cushioning in the area gets affected.

Here's a look at some of the most common issues causing joints to become inflamed and painful.

Arthritis

Arthritis, despite being very common, isn't well-understood. It's not a single disease but a name given to group of about 200 problems that affect the joints. The root cause behind all of these problems is inflammation of the joints.

Arthritis can affect people of all ages but is most common in women and older individuals. The common symptoms that you can experience during arthritis are pain, swelling, decreased mobility and stiffness. Symptoms can range from mild and moderate to severe. As arthritis worsens, you may find doing everyday tasks a nuisance. Inability to climb the stairs or bend down are common symptoms of progressed arthritis.

Osteoarthritis is arthritis that occurs when wear and tear of cartilage takes place. Being the most common type of arthritis, this problem is characterized by excessive pain and stiffness. As the cartilage wears away, there's no cushioning left for the bones. So, when you move, the bones run against each other and this friction causes the feeling of discomfort.

If the problem persists, the condition can get worse and joint strength is lost. The risk factors for this problem are obesity, age and any previous injury. Anyone with a family history of osteoarthritis is also likely to get it at some point in their life.

Arthritis can impact any set of joints, but its effects are felt most in the hips, knees, neck, back or the hands.

Another example is rheumatoid arthritis which is a kind of autoimmune disease. In this condition, inflammation increases in the body which causes joint damage and pain. Risk factors include genetic and environmental reasons.

For example, smoking is a risk factor that can cause rheumatoid arthritis in specific people who have a particular gene. The aim of medication that is given for treating this disease is to increase mobility and reduce stiffness.

Arthritis is diagnosed by a physician by doing blood testing and taking some imaging scans. If the problem gets bad, an orthopedic surgeon performs joint replacement surgery. Arthritis may also affect other parts of the body when it progresses, so other specialists like dentists and ophthalmologists may also be needed.

Gout

While the knees, neck and shoulders are spots more susceptible to joint pain, gout presents itself in the big toe of the foot. It's a very common type of arthritis that causes stiffness in the area which is accompanied by excessive swelling and intense pain. While it's common in men, women who have reached menopause also become more susceptible to gout.

The cause of this joint problem is the deposition of uric acid in the blood stream. This could be due to two reasons; either there is too much uric acid production or the kidney is not able to efficiently remove uric acid from the body. Inflammation, resulting from excess of uric acid crystals in the blood, is the prime cause of this problem.

Gout attacks are specific and quick, mostly occurring in the middle of the night. Medication is used to treat gout problems. It is used for reducing the symptoms and preventing future attacks. Since worsening of gout can also cause kidney stones, medication is used to prevent the situation from getting any more complex.

Bursitis

Bursitis is an inflammatory condition that affects the bursa. The bursa is a sac that is filled with fluid, present between the skin and the joints. As it is present above the joints, it acts as a cushioning agent between bones and tendons.

Common symptoms associated with bursitis are swelling and tenderness. Bursitis mostly occurs in elbows, knees, hips, knees and shoulders but other areas in the body can also get affected.

Bursas become inflamed when there is a repetitive movement or injury. If you indulge in any sports or physical activity where you are performing repetitive activities on daily basis, your chances of getting bursitis increase.

For example, if you bowl every day, you may get elbow bursitis. People who spend a lot of time on their knees such as gardeners are also prime victims of knee bursitis. Sometimes, bursitis may even be caused as a development in another arthritis condition such as gout.

Bursitis can also be treated at home. Easy treatment methods for bursitis are forming a cold pack or resting the area. Also, painkillers such as paracetamol can also help speed up the recovery process. Although the pain goes away in a few weeks, swelling lasts for a longer time.

To prevent bursitis, it is important that you wear knee pads when you are playing and always warm up before exercising. If your symptoms are not getting better at home even after 10 to 14 days of treatment, then seek medical help.

Injuries Caused by Repetitive Movement

Repetitive motion or stress injuries could be permanent or temporary injuries that cause damage to the nerves, tendons or ligaments. These injuries occur when you are doing the same thing over and over again.

For example, if you are playing a sport in which you do the same motion repetitively, then you are likely to suffer from a joint condition.

Carpel tunnel syndrome is a common form of such injury. It is caused by a disorder of tunnel that runs from the forearm to the wrist. When the ligaments and tendons in this area get compressed, swelling and pain are experienced. This type of repetitive movement injury is common in people who type on computer keyboards on daily basis.

This injury can cause a lot of pain. Numbness and lack of motion is also associated with this joint problem. If it persists, over time, the sufferer loses flexibility in the region. If treatment is not done, the end result is complete loss of function.

Of the two hands, the dominant hand is more prone to this problem and women are three times more likely to get carpal tunnel syndrome as compared to men. People suffering from wrist trauma or diabetes are also at a greater risk of getting this problem.

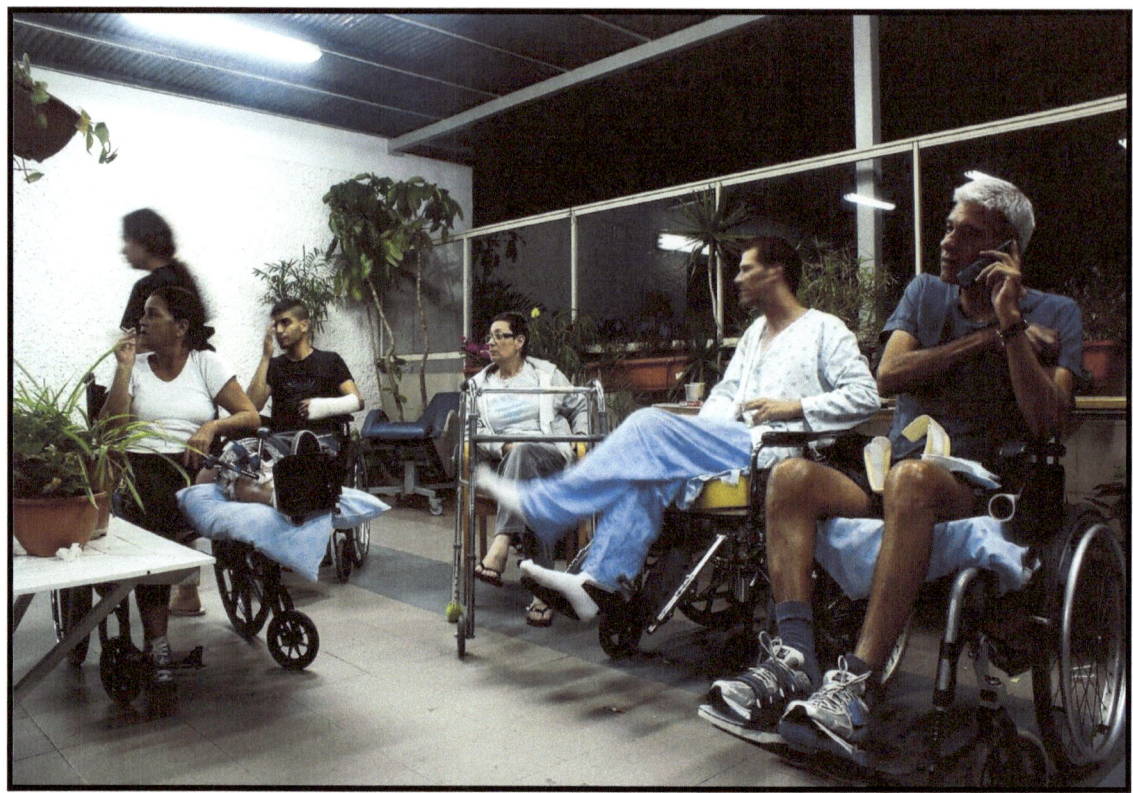

Rehabilitation programs for repetitive movement injury includes occupational therapy and pain management techniques. Heat and cold applications at home can also help. Exercising the affected area helps to strengthen it and prevent any complete loss of mobility. Primary care doctors, medicine doctors, sports doctors and orthopedic surgeons are involved in treatment of repetitive movement injuries. It is always best to get help before the condition gets any worse.

CHAPTER 3

GOOD JOINT HEALTH THROUGH EXERCISE

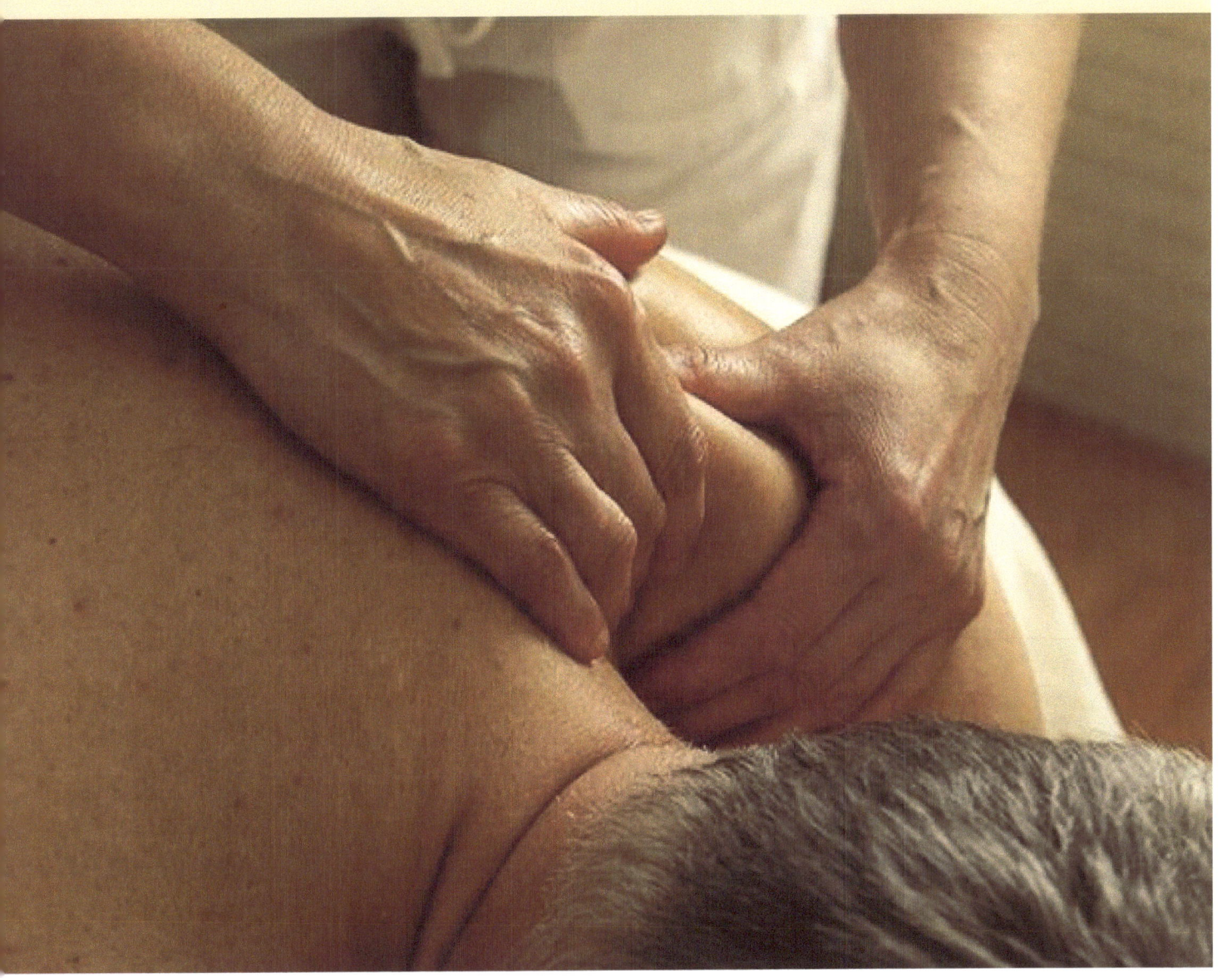

Chapter 3

Good Joint Health Through Exercise

To prevent joint damage and increase joint strength, exercise is very important. To preserve your joint health, you need to work on certain aspects of exercise that will keep your joints mobile, and minimize damage brought on by age or other factors. Here's what you need to keep in mind when doing so.

Increasing Flexibility and Range of Motion

The range of motion of a joint refers to the positions in which the joint can move. Joints prone to damage will reduce the range of motion and joint mobility. As such you need to follow an exercise program with three important components; endurance training, range of motion, and strengthening exercises. These exercises will help prevent the joint from any future damage or degradation.

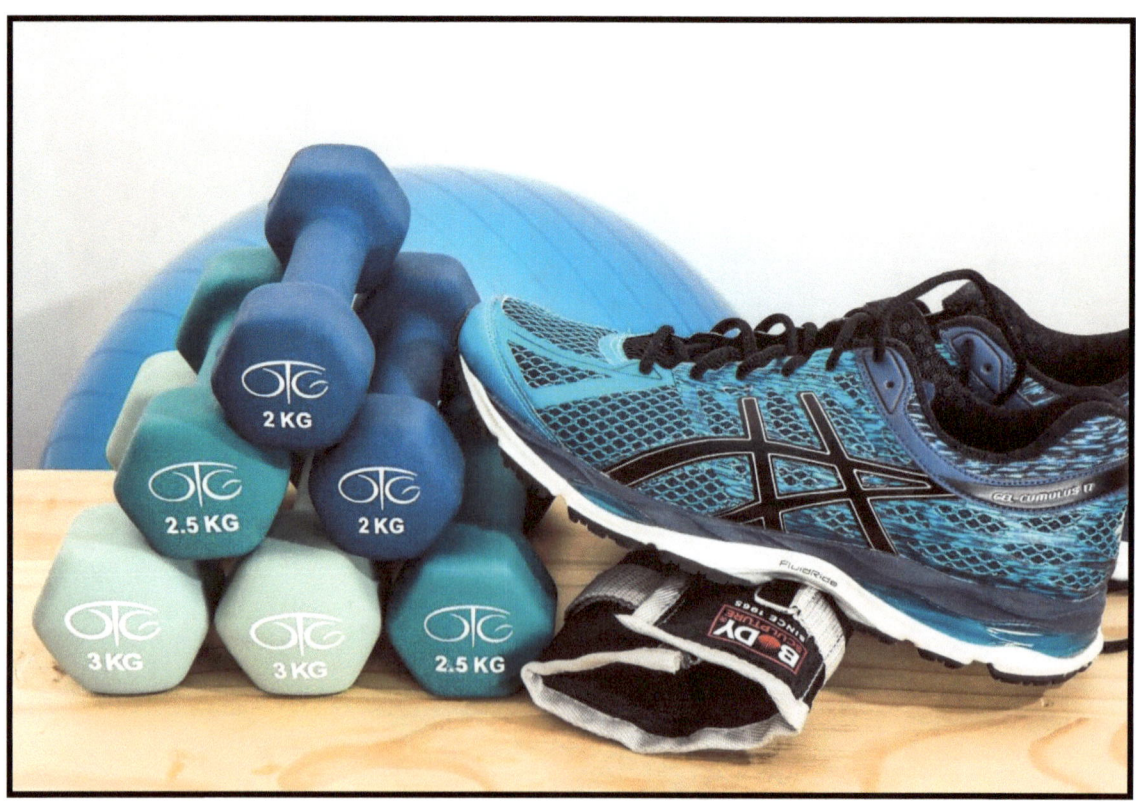

Exercises help to maintain optimum joint movement and increase flexibility. When you work out, your weight is also kept in check which further contributes to reducing the risks associated with arthritis and other joint-related conditions.

Flexibility exercises keep the cartilage strong and increase cushioning for the bones. The exercises are stretches that help increase elasticity of muscles while range of motion workouts lower the stiffness in joints.

An easy stretching exercise is stretching your legs while you are in bed. Patients of rheumatoid arthritis cannot get out of bed in the morning due to RA flares. They can get rid of them by performing leg stretches for 10 minutes.

In a hamstring stretch, you must sit up and extend your right leg in front of you. Bend the other leg and keep your left foot on the bed. Now, slide your hands on the right side and you will feel a stretch in the backside of your leg. Hold this position for 30 seconds to a minute and then do the same on the left leg.

Strengthen Your Core to Make Daily Tasks Easier

You may not want to be too obsessed with getting a six pack while you suffer from joint immobility, but core exercises are important nevertheless. Abdominal and back strength are important for doing daily chores like lifting a grocery bag or sitting at your desk working.

A very easy exercise for strengthening your core is the Knee Fold Tuck. For this exercise, sit on the floor and bend your knees. Keep a ball between your legs and squeeze it. Lift your knees until the shins and floor are parallel to each other. Then, start pulling your knees towards your shoulders and take them back to original position. Do this 10 to 15 times.

Climbing Rope is another strengthening exercise in which you sit with your legs extended. Your feet must be in a V position. Roll your spine in a C shape and then lift your arms. Your arms must mimic the motion of climbing a rope. As you reach, twist your body slightly. Do a total of 40 reaches with 20 of each arm. This will help keep your back and abdomen strong. It will also increase your arm strength and increase flexibility.

Planks are the best exercises for your core. They tighten the abdominal muscles and keep your back strong. Get into plank position and tighten your abs. Pull your right knee in and rotate is clockwise first and then counter clockwise. Do the same with the leg knee. Repeat the same step five times on both knees.

Variety is Key to a Balanced Body

Variety is the key when it comes to exercises. You must have diversity in your workouts so that all parts of the body get equal benefits. There are five elements of fitness; stretching, balance training, core exercises, aerobic exercises and strength training. If you're working out on a daily basis, you might get comfortable with one exercise and get into a habit of doing the same one every day. This might keep you comfortable but won't benefit you much in the other four areas.

When you do the same thing every day, your body gets used to it and it's no longer a challenge for your muscular or nervous system. It takes your body about six to eight weeks to get accustomed to a work out. After that, it no longer remains a challenge for the body to perform this exercise.

So, you need to bring some variety into your exercise routine to get added benefits. Same goes for joint exercises. And, if you keep working the same joint all the time, it can undergo degradation too. This, in itself, becomes a kind of overuse for the same joints so you need a well-tailored exercise plan that includes all joints.

Specific Exercises for Common Joints

Here's a rundown of some specific exercises focused on specific joint or parts.

Neck

The easiest exercise for the neck is to slowly drop your neck until your chin reaches the chest level. Keep the neck in this position for 5 to 10 seconds and then return to the original position. Tilt your head slightly back and remain in this position for 10 seconds. Do this stretch five times in each direction. Do the same side to side. It will help increase flexibility in the region and increase movement.

Another exercise is to sit in a chair in a good posture and rotate your neck. Firstly, turn your head to the right side and remain in this position for 10 seconds, then go back to the center and turn to the left. Hold the position in both sides for 10 seconds. You'll feel your neck muscles relax, relieve some tension while your joints in the area benefit too.

Shoulders

To prevent or minimize shoulder pain, try the arm across chest stretch. Holding you right arm out, take it across your chest to the left. Place your left hand just behind your right elbow and give your right arm a gentle stretch. Hold for 10 seconds. The point is to stretch your arm across the chest without feeling pain. Repeat on other side.

Another exercise is the chest expansion where you stand in a good posture and hold an exercise band. Now, take your arms back until your shoulder blades touch and hold the position for 5 to 10 seconds. Repeat 5-6 times to strengthen shoulders or relieve shoulder pain. The same will also help increase flexibility in the region.

Back

Pelvic Tilt is a back exercise in which you lie on the floor and bend your knees. Then, keeping your arms at your side, tighten your abdominal muscles. Do not use your butt or legs to pull your abdomen towards the spine. You will feel your pelvis moving up but not leaving the floor. Stay in this position for 5 seconds and then relax. Do 10 reps.

Hands and Wrists

An easy exercise is to make a fist. Slowly, bend your hand and keep your thumb on the outside. Open the hand again and straighten the fingers. Repeat for a minute or two with each hand.

Another exercise is to keep your hand open straight and then bend your thumb. Bend all your fingers towards the palm, one by one, and hold in that position for a few seconds. Do the same on the left hand.

Knees

Lie on the floor and bend both your legs. Lift one leg and bring your knee towards the chest. Keep your hands linked behind your thigh and slowly straighten the leg. Now, pull your straightened leg backwards and you will feel a stretch. Remain in this position for 30 seconds.

You can also do a half squat, in which you stand straight and then bend your knees to reach a half-sitting position. In leg stretch, sit with both legs straight in front of you on the floor or bed and bend one knee. Once you feel the stretch, hold in that position for 10 seconds and then straighten your leg slowly.

Be especially careful when performing knee exercises to maintain proper balance, if your knees are not up to doing squats and lunges, skip these for easier exercises.

CHAPTER 4

THE ROLE OF DIET IN JOINT HEALTH

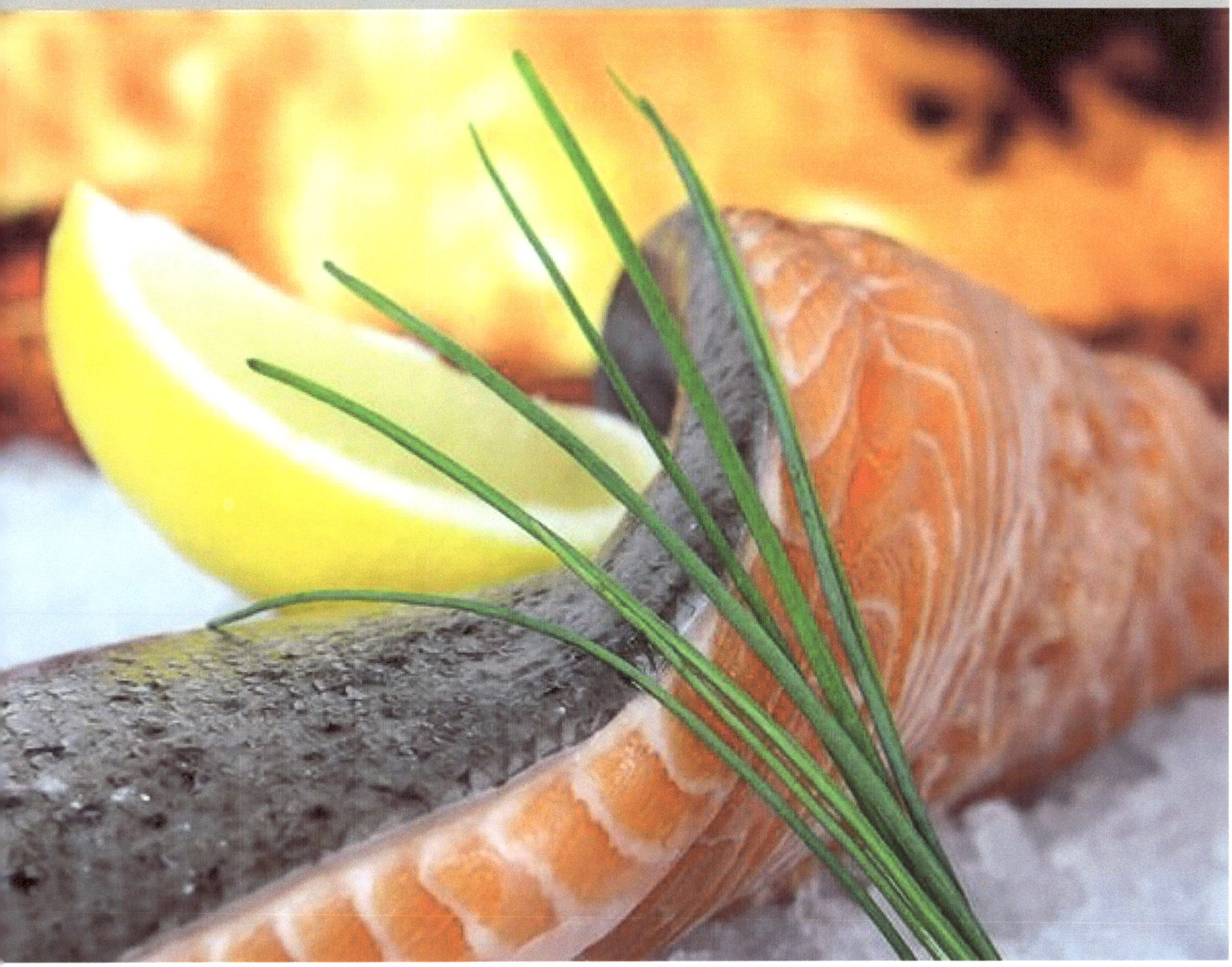

Chapter 4

The Role of Diet in Joint Health

If you don't lead a healthy life with a balanced diet, health issues will catch up with you sooner than you'd like. There's always room for improvement and you can start making changes in your diet at any point in life. A joint-healthy diet helps keep away pain, stiffness and reduced mobility.

Nourish Your Joints with Good Nutrition

The food you eat contains different nutrients such as fats, proteins, fiber, vitamins and carbohydrates. The two most important nutrients for joint health are minerals and vitamins.

The most notable among these is perhaps calcium which keeps your bones strong and can prevent osteoporosis. But while many people give calcium the credits it deserves for bone and joint health, they often forget about magnesium. However, the truth is that calcium needs to be paired with magnesium, and even vitamin D to be most effective.

You need to have a good balance of all three as each is dependent on the other for optimal performance. For instance, while calcium promotes bone density, magnesium assists the transport of calcium across cell membranes. At the same time, magnesium promotes enzymes that convert vitamin D to its active form, which, in turn helps the body absorb calcium better.

Magnesium also plays a role in strengthening bones and maintaining cartilage. It also regulates nerve and muscle function, ensuring that everything is under control. Studies have shown that magnesium prevents degradation of bones and increases bone density. It's also been found to be effective against postmenopausal osteoporosis.

People with joint issues often suffer from low levels of vitamin D as well. According to studies, Vitamin D seems to ward off conditions like osteomalacia or soft bones, or osteoporosis, resulting in loss of bone mass. Supplementing well with this vitamin may help you take better care of your bones and joints.

Another vitamin that deserves attention in this area is vitamin C. as one of the most powerful antioxidants, it can help prevent oxidative stress in the body. Oxidative stress also harms the synovial membrane in joints causing the synovial fluid to leak, compromising joint lubrication. Here vitamin C can provide cushion and lubrication to the area by preventing oxidative damage.

Best Foods for Good Joint Health

Naturally, the best foods for joint health will include these aforementioned nutrients along with others. If you already suffer from joint-related conditions, then altering your diet may actually help reduce your painful or discomforting issues.

For instance, there are some foods that can actually help reduce the effects of arthritis and also relieve pain. Many patients suffering from arthritis admit that changes in their diet plan have helped reduce the severity of their symptoms.

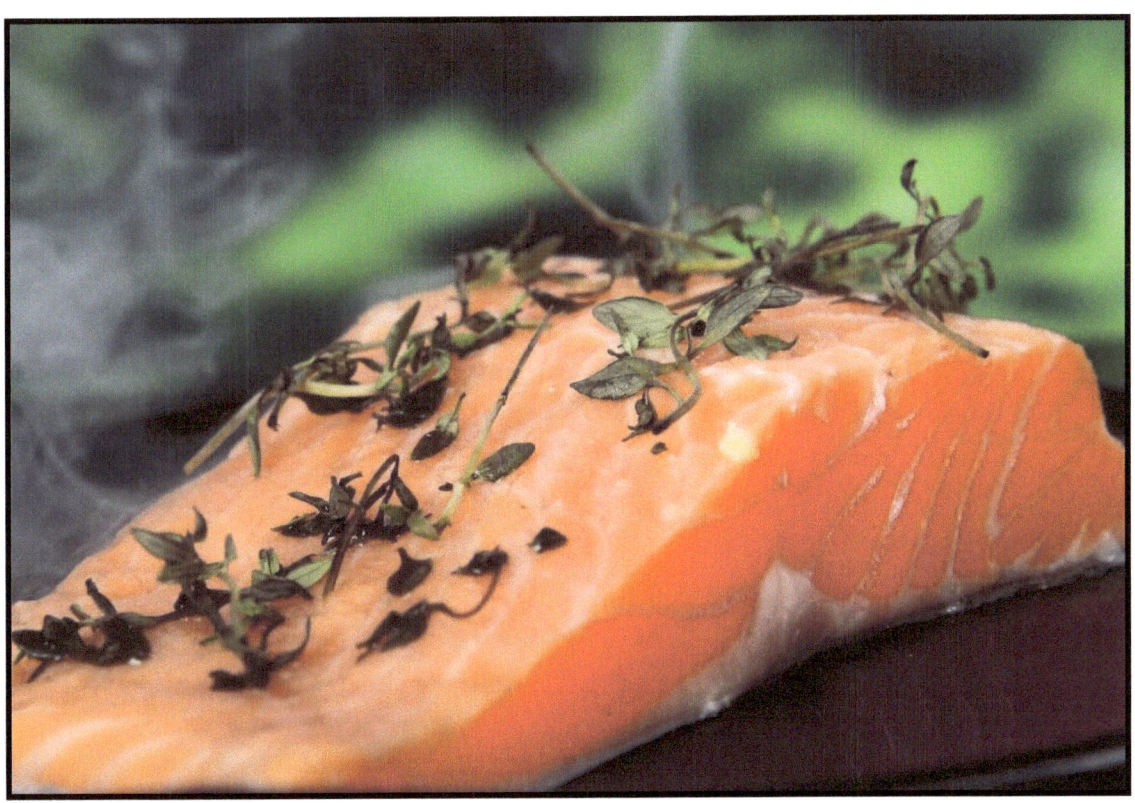

One of the best foods to eat if you have painful or inflamed joints is fatty fish. Salmon and sardines are rich in omega 3 fatty acids. Omega 3s reduce inflammation in the body and it has been found that in the presence of this fatty acid, the amount of inflammatory mediators is also low in the body.

Incorporating Omega 3s in your diet will reduce morning stiffness, provide pain-relief and cool down your body. These fatty acids are especially helpful for people with rheumatoid arthritis.

Garlic is also very important for people suffering from painful joints. Its immune strengthening properties make cells stronger and can target inflammation as well. By lowering the amount of inflammatory markers in the body, garlic helps lessen the pain associated with arthritis and similar conditions.

Likewise, ginger is also very effective in reducing pain from knee arthritis. A very easy way to incorporate these two foods in your diet is to make a garlic ginger paste and use it for flavoring in your meals.

Broccoli is not only effective for keeping your weight in check but also great for joint health. It's involved in blocking a certain type of cell that accelerates the progression of rheumatoid arthritis. Walnuts are also anti-inflammatory in their effect and they may even reduce the need for painkillers. If you love berries, then you are in luck because berries also reduce inflammatory markers associated with arthritis. Whether it's black berries or strawberries, all kinds are great for joint health.

Spinach is another green that helps promote joint health. Spinach is a powerful green vegetable that helps prevent the progression of osteoarthritis. At the same time, it also improves cartilage health and reduces inflammatory agents that cause rheumatoid arthritis. Another fruit for fighting joint pain is Grapes. The outer covering of grapes contains resveratrol, which has antioxidant properties. Grapes also slow down the thickening of joints and block the production of cells causing rheumatoid arthritis. You can also prepare your meals in olive oil to promote the health of your joints.

Avoid These Foods!

There are some foods that you need to avoid in order to prevent progression or worsening of joint pains. Firstly, fried foods and processed edibles are a huge No for anyone with painful joints. These foods can significantly decrease the body's immunity and cause inflammation.

When you cut down the intake of such foods, the body's natural defense system gets restored. Instead of eating frozen foods, cook at home and try to go for greens and fruits. Even foods cooked at high temperatures can make your body more prone to arthritis, so opt for more suitable recipes.

AGE or Advanced Glycation End Product, as they increase in the body, can cause inflammation. These are produced when you eat grilled or heated foods. The body activates cytokines that cause inflammation in response, to fight these compounds. As a result of that, the overall level of inflammation increases in the body causing a risk of joint pain or deterioration. Cut down on these foods so that blood AGE levels can be low.

You might love nibbling on cheese slices but this isn't healthy for your joints. Dairy products contribute to joint deterioration due to their protein content. Proteins present in dairy products can irritate the surrounding tissue of joints in many people. You can get the same proteins from other sources without the side effects, so it's advised to switch to a restricted dairy diet.

Corn oil is present in many snacks and some baked goods too. It gives a pleasant taste to food but can trigger inflammatory markers to go in action and increases the risk of joint pain. This is because corn oil is rich in Omega 6 fatty acids. Instead of eating omega 6s, you can try using oils rich in Omega 3s, such as olive oil and flaxseed oil.

Some cuts of red meat can also exacerbate inflammation as they are rich in saturated fats. Also, excessive consumption of red meat can cause obesity which is another factor contributing to joint pain. Experts say that gluten can also cause inflammation in people who are already suffering from an autoimmune disease such as rheumatoid arthritis.

Although alcohol doesn't really count as food, increased intake can lead to deterioration of joint health. A controlled amount of alcohol can actually prevent RA but the problem begins when you start drinking too much of it.

Overconsumption of alcohol leads to production of a protein called C - reactive protein which is a signal for inflammation. So, it can worsen the cases of rheumatoid arthritis. Balancing your diet is the first step towards improving joint health.

CHAPTER 5

HOW WEIGHT AFFECTS JOINTS

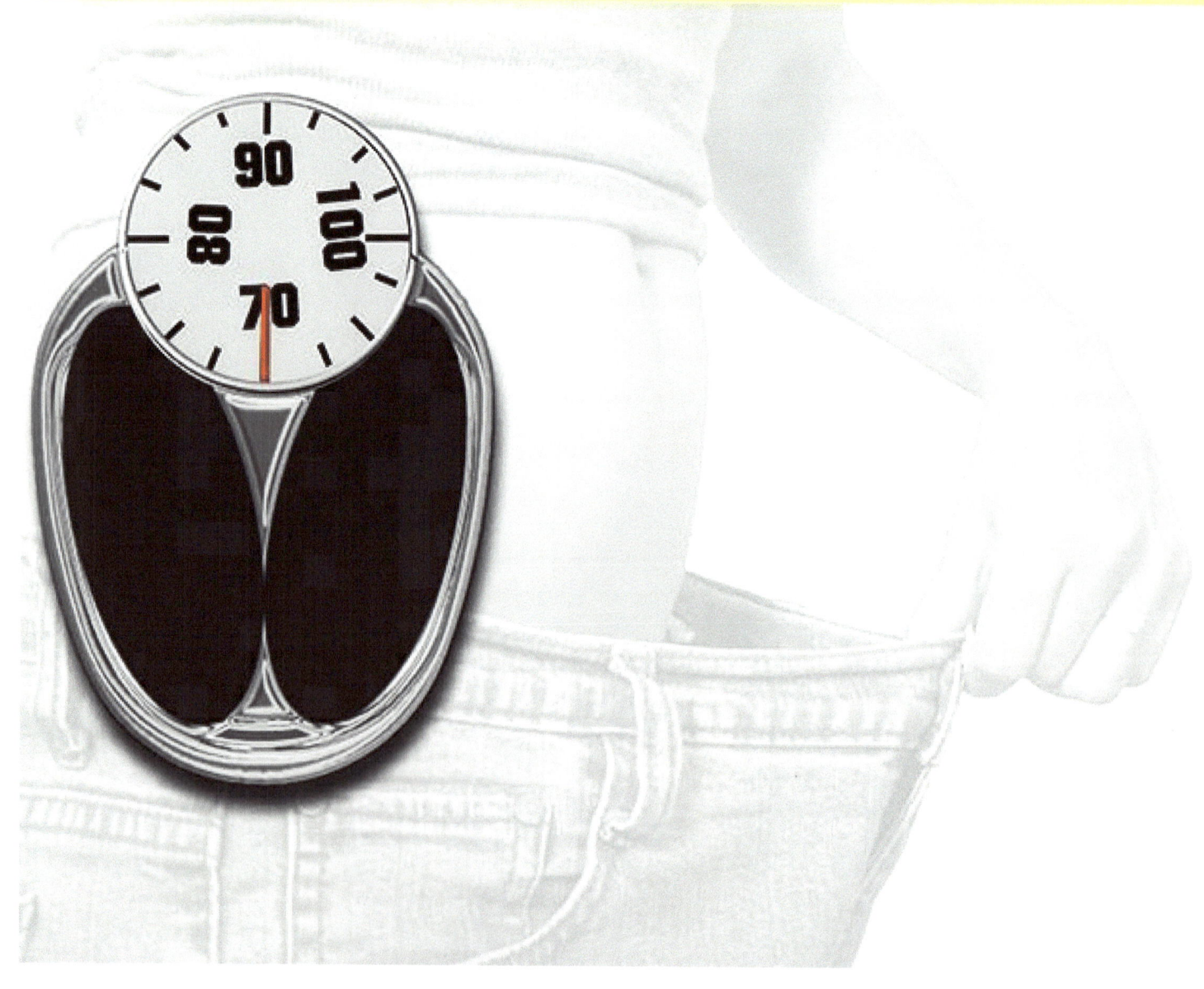

Chapter 5

How Weight Affects Joints

So now that you know that one of the factors affecting joint health is lack of physical activity, what do you do about it? Well, you naturally start off with some form of exercise to improve joint flexibility and range of motion. But at the same time, you also have to watch your weight.

When your body becomes too heavy to be supported by your joints and bones, problems start to arise. As such, you need to exercise and eat right to keep your body at an optimal weight.

Weight and How It Affects Joints

If you have a sensation of pain when walking for a while or climbing up the stairs and are worried because it runs in the family, then you should take a look at your weight. Being overweight increases your chances of getting osteoarthritis. As mentioned earlier, this condition is caused by the wear and tear in joints and is the most common form of bone degradation.

When you're overweight, there's extra stress on the joints that bears your weight. The most common of these joints is the knee joint and it's the first one to get affected by excess weight. The second reason why weight is detrimental for joints is that as your weight increases, the inflammatory markers in the body also increase. This further causes joint deterioration in other places such as your hands and neck.

The extra pounds in your body stressing your joints can lead to degeneration of cartilage and joint damage. In cases of osteoporosis, being overweight also increases the rate of bone degeneration. By shedding weight, you can protect your joints from extra stress and any further damage. Experts suggest that you should lose about 10% of your body weight and then see if the symptoms improve.

If they do, then it's your weight causing the problems in the first place. Obesity further reduces any physical activity which becomes another cause for joint issues in the long run. And if you already suffer from an extreme case of arthritis, high endurance exercise can also damage to your joints.

So, it's important to get guidance from an expert about the kind of exercises you can and should do. In osteoarthritis, sitting for extended periods of time causes stress on the joints and worsens the pain. If you have an office job, make a habit to take a walk or do short exercises after every hour.

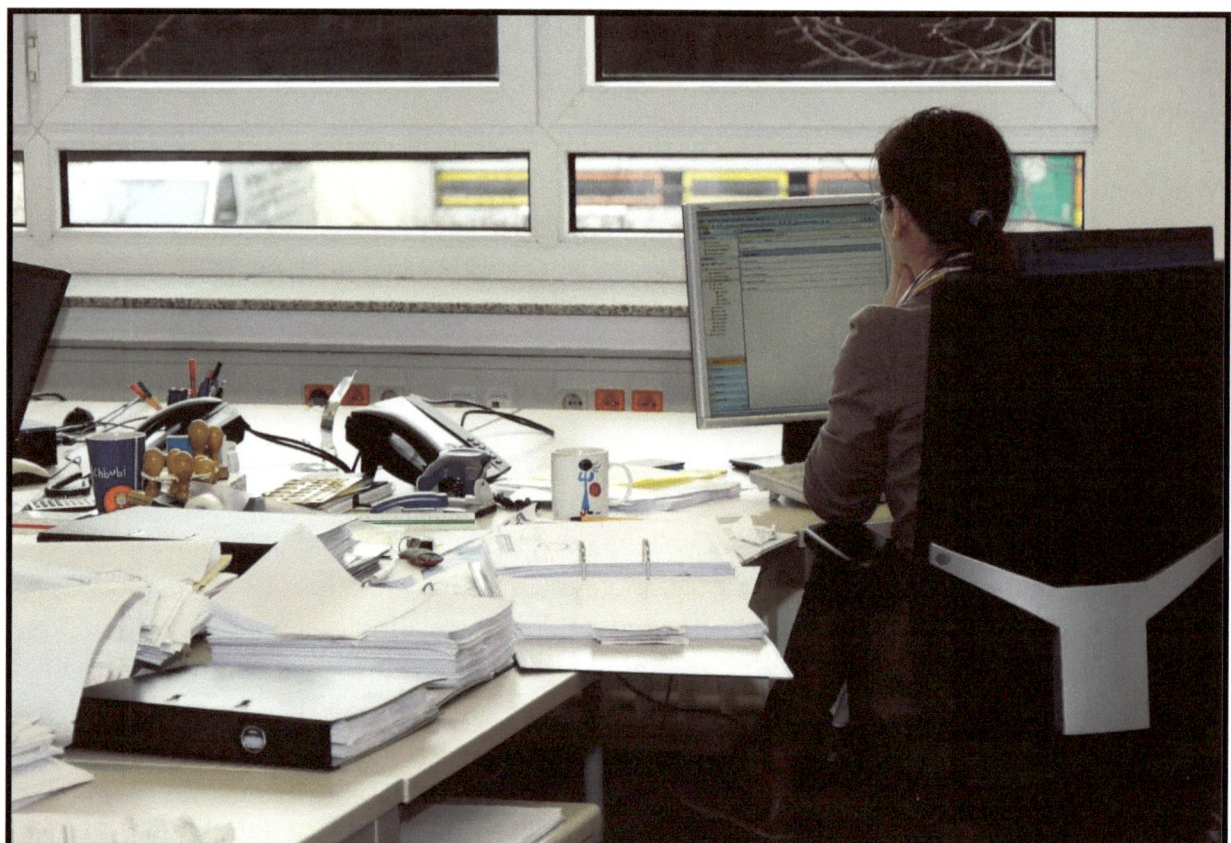

Reduce Stress on Joints – Reduce the Pain

Weight loss is a great way to reduce stress on your joints. On average, the amount of pressure or stress on your knees is 1 ½ times that of your body weight. So, if you weigh 300 pounds, you are putting 450 pounds of stress on your knees. This is when you are in standing position. As the incline increases, the stress increases too.

As such, when you climb stairs, there's more stress on your knees. If your knees are extremely close to the ground, like when you tie a shoelace, the weight increases to three or four times of your body weight.

Experts say that just a 10-pound increase in weight increases 30 to 40 pounds of stress on your joints. The joints work fine while they are still young and healthy but after an extended period of time, they give up.

So just imagine that if you lose weight, how much stress you'll be able to reduce on your knees. When you're young, the body's cells proliferate at a considerable rate. With age, this process slows down so the damaged cells don't get repaired as quickly as they did during your youth.

So start slow and you'll be able to lose the extra pounds very easily. Physical activity in the form of exercise is a proven way of slowing the progression of arthritis. Just like any machine, the body wears away if it is not being used properly. So, put your muscles and joints to use so that they do not erode away, but do it sensibly so that you don't overuse them and cause further damage. It ends up being a balancing act as far as what is optimal for your joints.

Every pound you lose represents about 3500 calories. So, if you're hoping to lose one pound in a week, you need to burn about 500 more calories per day than you consume. The exercise plan you follow must at least help you lose those 500 calories in a day. Another way to do it is to reduce the number of calories you eat by 250 calories per day and burn off an additional 250 calories through exercising for a total of 500 fewer calories per day.

Along with exercise, you also need to focus on your diet. Even if you're young and not arthritic, it's essential that you watch your weight to dodge this disease in a few years' time.

Good Posture – Less Pain

It's a basic rule of thumb that good posture can save you from a lot of pain. Improper posture often becomes the cause of back pain and knee pain. Standing up straight is a good way to keep your knees, legs and back safe from stress.

When you slouch, you increase the stress on your joints. As mentioned above, the closer your knees are to the ground, the more stress they bear. So when you stand, make sure there is no incline and you are straight to minimize stress on your knee joint.

Whatever you do, it's important to have proper posture to keep your back muscles and knee joint safe. For example, if you are a student and you need to hold your backpack for a long time, sling it over both your shoulders rather than just one. This divides the stress instead of concentrating it only on one side.

Likewise, if you carry a handbag, keep changing your arms after a few minutes. Don't sling it only on one shoulder for a long time as that can damage the hinge joints in the region.

Proper posture is essential because it also keeps your bones and joints aligned. When you have a bad posture, this alignment gets disturbed and causes the joints to rub against each other. When this keeps happening over time, wear and tear starts to take place.

Your spine takes the stress and starts presenting issues. If you have a kind of job where you need to sit for many hours, make sure you have proper posture. Shoulders should be over hips and you should have good lower back support. Your computer screen should be at eye level so that you don't have to put strain on your neck to look at the screen. Keep your elbows at 90 degrees and the pens or other things you may need should be in easy reach.

When you have to tie your shoe lace, sit on a chair and keep your foot on the opposite knee. In this way, you won't have to bend too far down. Bending too far increases stress on your joints. So, the idea behind proper posture and exercise is not only to keep joints healthy but also to slow down the degradation process.

CHAPTER 6

EASING JOINT PAIN WITH HOME REMEDIES

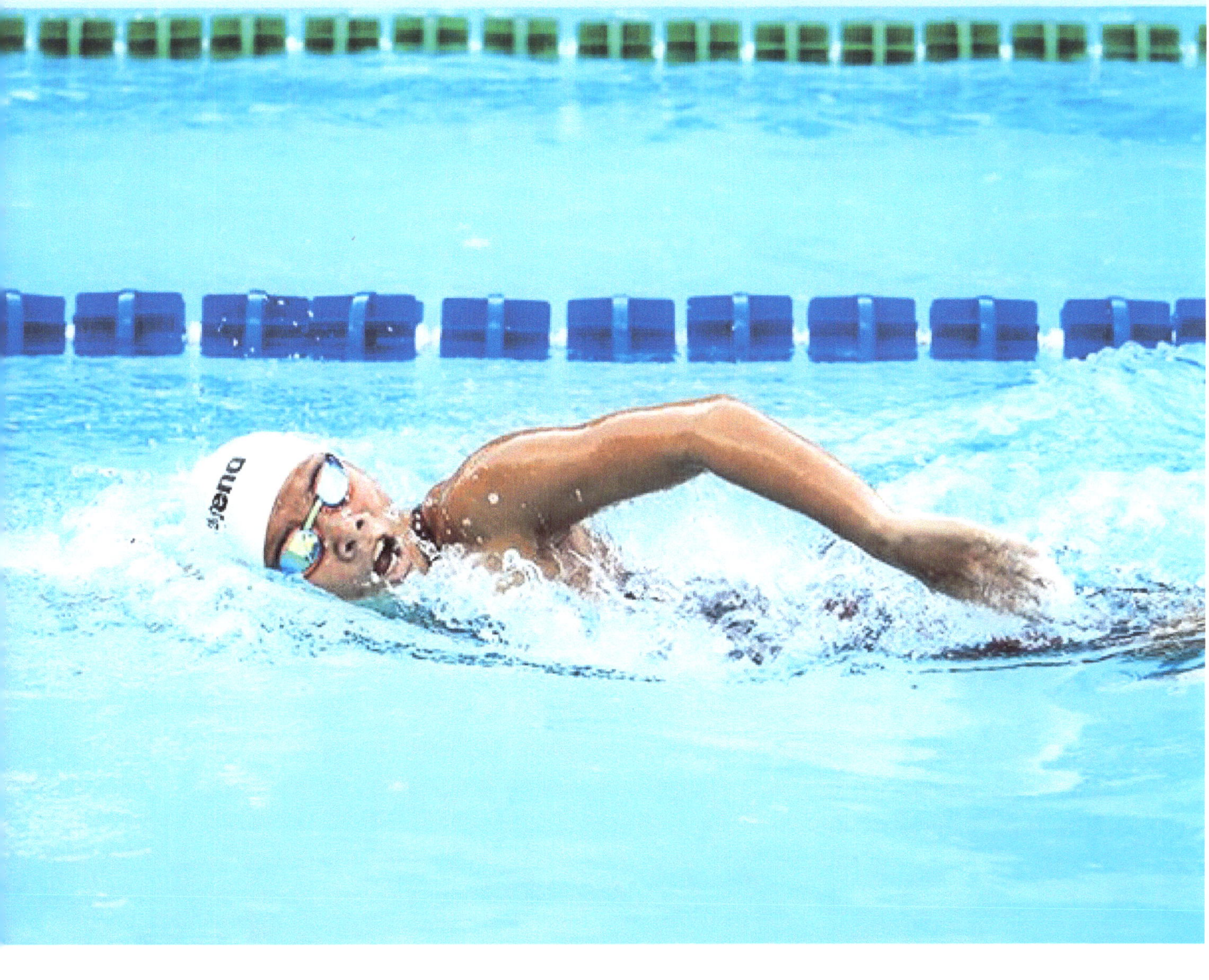

Chapter 6

Easing Joint Pain with Home Remedies

Oftentimes, doctors prescribe painkillers and anti-inflammatory drugs for joint pain. But if you're someone concerned about the side effects of medication, as I was mentioned in the Introduction, you may just wish to use some tried-and-true home remedies instead. Where the pain isn't too bad or too frequent, you may be able to get relief from these simple home remedies. These remedies are effective for treating joint pain in knees, neck, hips, ankles and lower back.

Epsom Salts

Epsom salts have been used traditionally for treating joint and muscle pains. These salts are rich in sulphates and magnesium, like many supplements used for treating joint pain. They can be administered topically as they are absorbed by the skin. These salts aid in relaxing the tensed regions of the body while keeping muscle spasms at minimum. You can simply add two cups of Epsom salts to your bath water and stay in it for about half an hour.

Or, you can make a compress of these salts and apply to the skin topically. For doing this, add two cups of Epsom salts in one gallon of water to form a dilute mixture. Then dip a towel or face cloth in this solution and apply to the affected area. Adding essential oils to the mixture can increase the benefits of this remedy.

Essential Oils

Essential oils are also great home remedies for joint pain. Lavender essential oil is extremely helpful in treating those conditions in which the pain is already present and is worsening. If you take an Epsom salt bath, simply add a few drops of lavender oil to the water. If the affected area is swollen and feels warm, this could be a case of bursitis. Apply peppermint oil to the area. The cooling menthol effect of this oil will reduce the swelling and inflammation.

Eucalyptus essential oil also reduces inflammation associated with arthritis and osteoarthritis. Along with that, it also helps prevent edema or fluid retention. Turmeric oils are not commonly available in many areas but they are helpful in reducing joint pain that occurs due to osteoarthritis, rheumatoid arthritis and bursitis. You can also add more turmeric to your daily meals to get maximum benefits.

Soaking the Sun

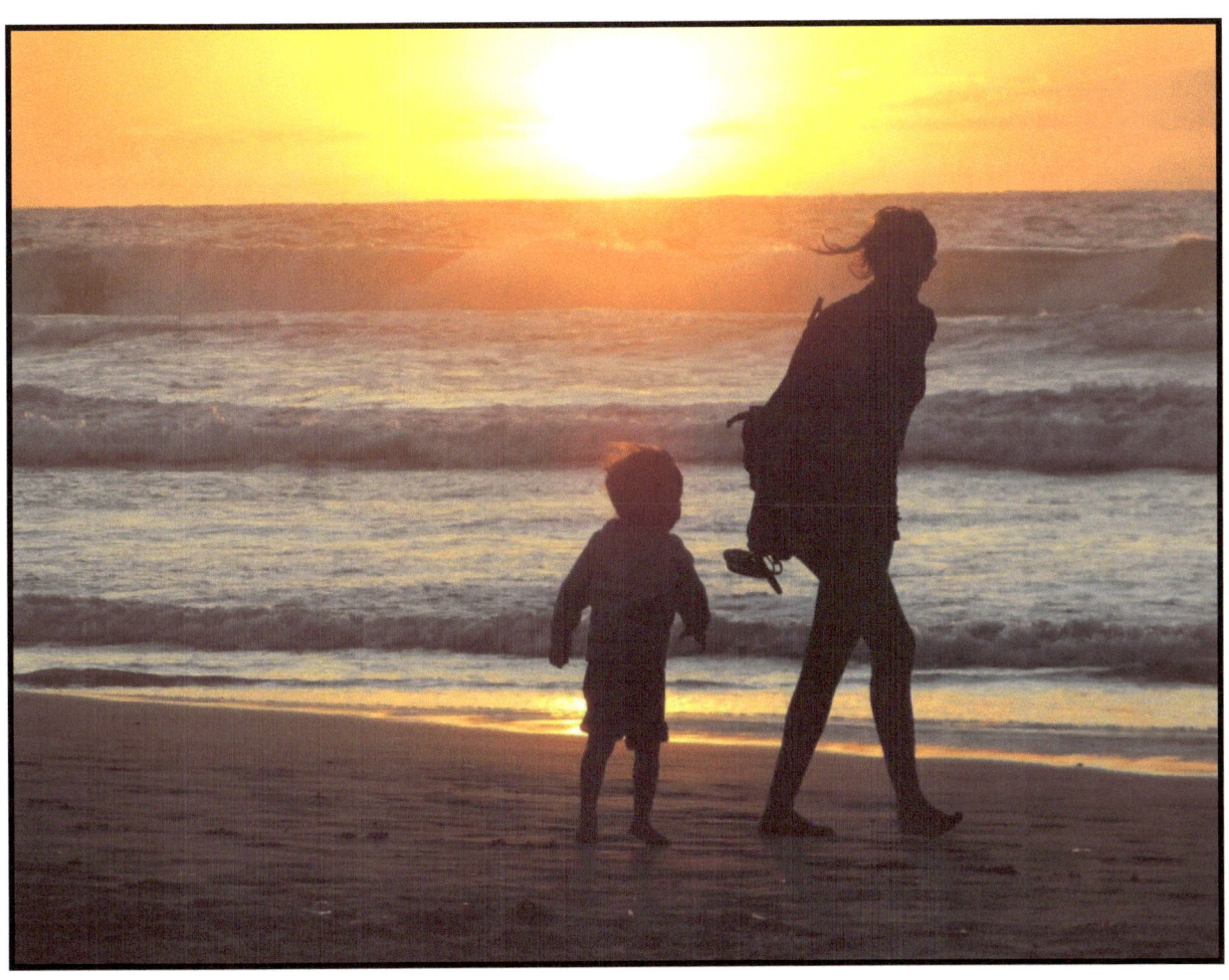

You'd be surprised at how helpful a good sun bath can be in getting rid of pain. Many people with joint issues have such complaints because of lower levels of Vitamin D. Your body naturally produces Vitamin D when you go out in the sun.

Expose your body to the sun for 20 minutes three to four times a week. Even this much exposure is enough for your body to make enough Vitamin D. So whenever it's a nice day outside, take a walk by yourself or with a friend and do your joints (and the rest of your body for that matter) a huge favor.

Hot and Cold Packs

Hot and cold packs are probably the most accessible home remedy for joint pain. Both, hot and cold treatments can help relieve pain and stiffness. There are two types of hot treatments; dry and moist. Taking long warm showers will often relieve any stiffness in the joints. Take a warm shower in the morning to feel more energetic during the day.

You can also keep a heating pad on affected areas to loosen up your joints while you sleep. When heat reaches the damaged areas, it provides relief and soothes muscles along with joints.

Cold treatments are great for reducing inflammation and ridding the body of pain. Apply the ice pack to affected area for quick relief. These two methods are lifesavers when the pain gets worse.

Chamomile Tea Poultice

Chamomile tea can also reduce the pain associated with arthritis. It helps cool down the body and reduce inflammation. There are different inflammatory markers in the body that heat up the system and disturb the internal balance. This tea soothes everything and calms the immune system.

To make a poultice, take four chamomile tea bags and add them in a cup of boiling water. Steep and keep the cup covered for about 20 minutes. Then remove the tea bags from the cup and soak a clean face cloth in the cup. When soaked with the liquid, apply to the affected area and you'll feel instant relief.

Swimming

As odd as it may sound, swimming can actually help reduce the pain that comes with arthritis. It is also a good exercise for losing weight if you suffer from joint pain. High intensity exercise is almost impossible for someone who has painful joints. Instead, exercising in water is easier as it bears less weight.

Not only does swimming reduce pain, it also increases flexibility in the hip region. In addition, it strengthens the hip muscles for increased mobility. In some areas, there are special swimming classes for people who suffer from arthritis. So, look around or go for a swim occasionally.

Soothing Music

If you love listening to music, you can actually use your hobby to get rid of the pain. Studies show that people who listened to soothing music had reduced arthritis pain as compared to people who were not given a music prescription. Besides, music also reduces the depression that comes with joint pain.

You don't necessarily have to listen to a particular genre or kind of music. The important thing is that you enjoy the music. If you like the music, your body activates several hormones that cause pain relief, acting as body's own natural pain killers. Listening to your favorite music for a bit every day can help take down the pain by several notches.

Acupuncture

Acupuncture is a Chinese treatment method that is thought to be effective in treating joint pain. In this method, thin needles are inserted at specific points in the body. These are particular pressure points and inserting needles in these points reroutes the energies in the body. At the same time, the normal balance of the body is restored. According to this treatment method, there are meridians or pathways in the body through which energy flows.

A total of 350 acupuncture points are present in the body for streamlining the flow of energy. Although there is no clear scientific explanation for this method, it is thought that acupuncture induces the body's natural painkillers to set into motion.

The World Health Organization recognizes this technique and it's considered to be useful for treating more than 100 conditions. Look for a licensed acupuncturist in your region or state. You can also learn the technique so that you can do it at home any time. All these remedies are sure to help you when you do not have medications at hand.

Walking

While this isn't exactly a remedy, it's a good way of keeping pain at bay. Walking barefoot reduces the pressure on joints by 12% as compared to the stress your joints feel when you walk in shoes. When you buy shoes, make sure that they mimic the natural arch of your foot. Lifting up your heel can cause stress on your joints. So, avoid wearing heels daily as this can cause damage to your joints. Wearing heels for extended period of time also increases the risk of joint damage.

CHAPTER 7

THE BEST SUPPLEMENTS FOR IMPROVED JOINT HEALTH

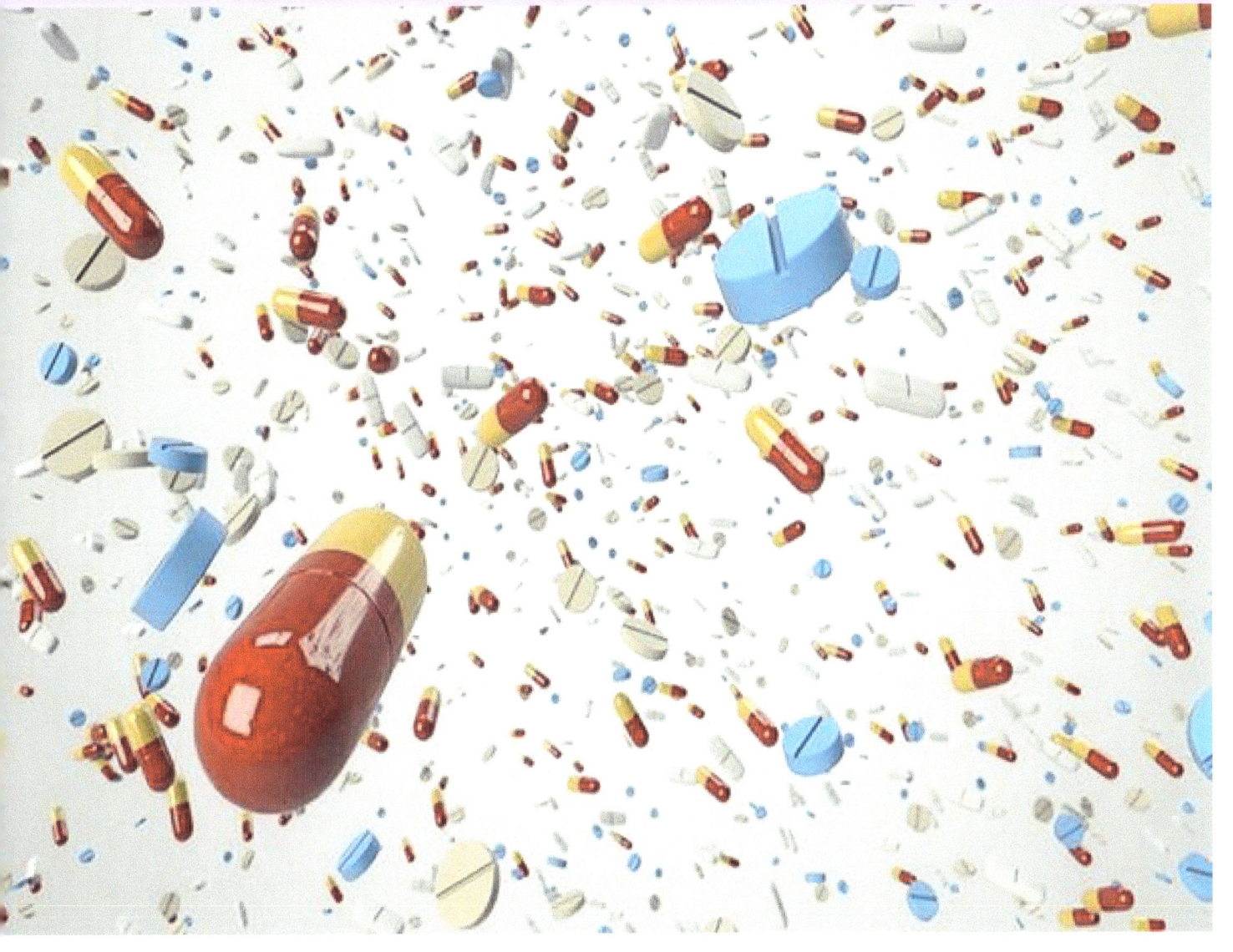

Chapter 7

The Best Supplements for Improved Joint Health

As you've seen previously, increased friction between joints leads to the sensation of pain and discomfort. While many resort to medication, (coming up in the next chapter) as the primary solution to the problem, supplements are also a popular alternative.

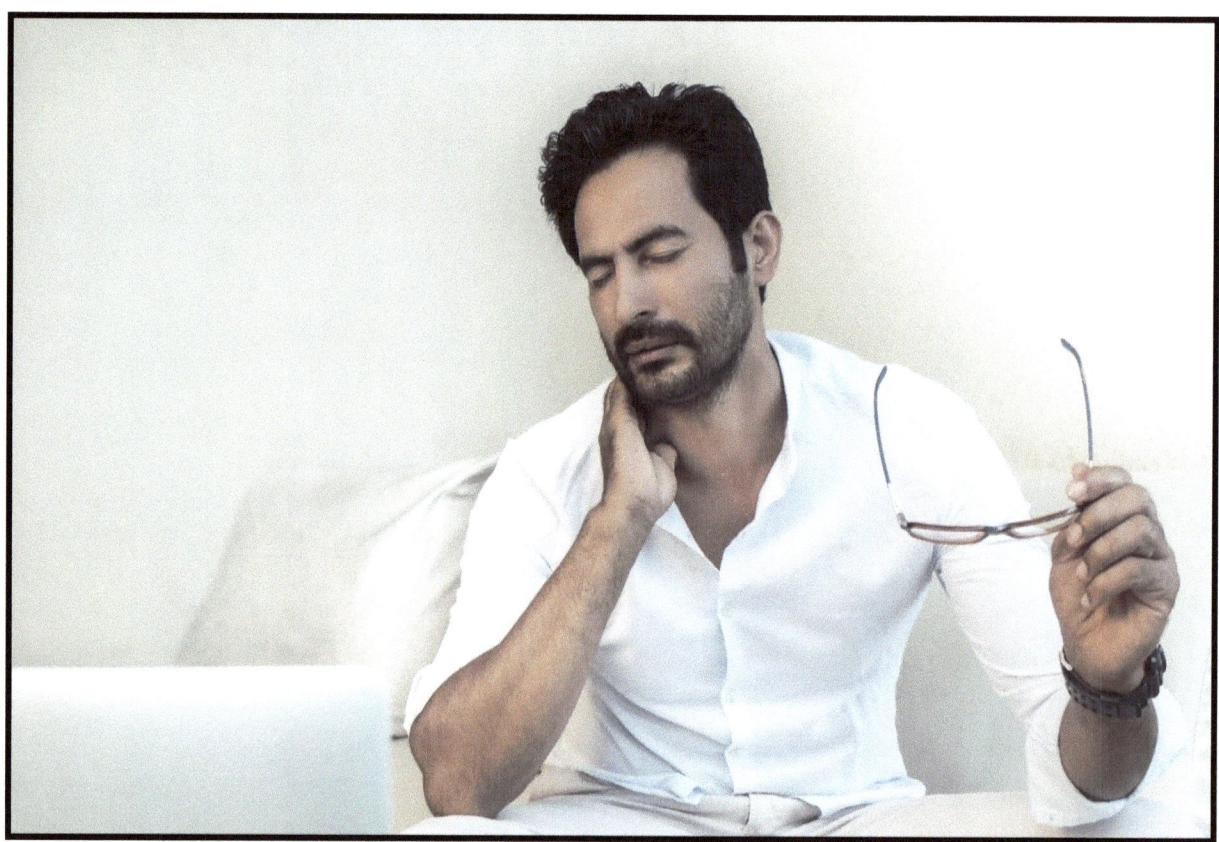

And while there is a plethora of supplements available, here we'll only look at some of the best in this category. These supplements have all been backed by scientific research and deemed most effective to addressing joint related issues.

Glucosamine

Glucosamine is a complex carbohydrate found in the body primarily in three different forms; glucosamine sulfate, glucosamine hydrochloride and N-acetyl-glucosamine. Among these, glucosamine sulfate is the most common form and is extracted from the outer covering of shellfish. To treat joint issues, this supplement may be used alone or combined with chondroitin or shark cartilage for added benefits.

The reason why this is considered beneficial for joint health is because it plays a vital role in the formation of cartilage. As you've already seen, cartilage thins and deteriorates with age. If anything, it needs help from supplementation to keep it healthy.

Evidence suggests that glucosamine helps in slowing down this process. It assists cartilage repair and formation by incorporating sulfur into the structure. Likewise, swelling also reduces in the presence of glucosamine. People suffering from hip or knee arthritis can sufficiently benefit from this supplement.

The pain-relieving effect of glucosamine lasts for about 3 months from usage so it may not exactly offer a long-term solution. Results may take a good 6-8 weeks to become noticeable but will likely be more effective than those achieved by using over-the-counter and prescription medication.

Chondroitin

Chondroitin naturally occurs in the body in bone and cartilage while supplementary chondroitin is extracted from animal cartilage.

Chondroitin is present in the form of chondroitin sulfate and is often administered alongside glucosamine. Its benefits are somewhat similar to that of glucosamine.

This supplement helps the cartilage retain water so that excess rubbing between bones may be prevented. At the same time, it also slows down the progression of osteoarthritis.

When used on its own or in association with other supplements, chondroitin improves the shock-absorbing ability of collagen protein. Also, it inhibits the functioning of enzyme that causes cartilage breakdown.

When used in conjunction with another supplement, hyaluronic acid, the two develop into a spring-like molecule. This improves the elasticity and strength of the cartilage. At the same time, chondroitin sulphate also signals the immune system to prevent cartilage breakdown by increasing collagen synthesis.

Chondroitin is especially beneficial for people with hand arthritis. Although it doesn't enhance grip strength or reduce the need for pain medication, it still alleviates morning stiffness in such individuals.

It can also serve as an alternative for NSAIDS for people who can't take them as no side effects of this supplement have been reported.

SAM-E

SAM-E is a compound that's naturally formed in the body. It plays a role in synthesis, activation and degradation of hormones, drugs and different proteins. The body produces chemicals that induce inflammatory responses to activate the immune system. SAM-E reduces the activity of these mediators to lower pain in joints.

In osteoarthritis, proteoglycan, which is a constituent of cartilage, doesn't get produced in sufficient amounts. SAM-E enhances the working of enzymes that form proteoglycan to reverse cartilage degradation. SAM-E also plays a role in reducing stiffness in joints. Consequently, mobility is improved. It's been seen to be very helpful in reversing the excessive fatigue and body pain associated with fibromyalgia.

Tendinitis, which refers to the inflammation of tendons in the body, is also treatable with the help of SAM-E. Bursa, a cushioning sac filled with fluid between tendons and bones, can be inflamed. This leads to swelling of the bursa and joint pain.

SAM-E is particularly helpful in reducing swelling and tenderness. Individuals suffering from chronic lower back pain due to weight or sports injury, can also benefit from this supplement.

Capsaicin

Capsaicin is a component of chili peppers. It's the constituent that causes a burning sensation in your mouth because it causes a sting when it comes in contact with any body tissue. The working of capsaicin is quite interesting as it relieves pain by affecting the nerve cells. It's used in form of a topical cream or patch.

It stimulates the activation of certain nerve receptors that are involved in causing itching or stinging sensation. Capsaicin keeps the receptors activated for a long period of time.

After some time, the receptors' ability to function is lost due to over-reception. So, these receptors also stop processing signals for pain induction. When used on regular basis, this supplement helps numb the sensation of pain by overusing the receptors.

Capsaicin is effective in relieving pain that is caused by rheumatoid arthritis, fibromyalgia and osteoarthritis. It is so effective that it can actually help lower the pain by 50% after just a month of usage. It also helps reduce pain which results from nerve damage as a result of diabetic neuropathy or HIV.

Curcumin

Curcumin is a chemical abundantly present in turmeric. Although turmeric is only used as a flavoring agent in cooking or to give color in cosmetics, it also has benefits for joint health. Curcumin reduces pain associated with rheumatoid arthritis and osteoarthritis.

When the bursa swells and causes irritation of joints, curcumin can also aid in reducing swelling and inflammation in the region for smooth cushioning and improved mobility. It blocks the enzymes that are involved in formation of inflammatory mediators in the body.

One of the targets of curcumin is COX-2, a mediator that is also target of many pain-relieving medicines. So, curcumin can act as an alternative to NSAIDS. Instead of reducing joint inflammation, this supplement actually prevents further inflammation. Patients suffering from knee osteoarthritis can benefit from this supplement. In some cases of rheumatoid arthritis, curcumin actually tends to be more effective than NSAIDS.

Omega 3s

Omega 3s are naturally found in fish oils and have been consumed for centuries for their benefits. One of the main benefits of omega 3s is pain relief.

The two important omega 3s for relieving pain are DHA (docosahexaenoic acid) and EPA (eicosapentaenoic acid). Omega 3s have shown most effectiveness in relieving pain due to rheumatoid arthritis. They don't reverse joint damage or play a role in synthesis of new cartilage. Instead, their only function is for pain relief.

When omega 3s are taken as supplements, they get converted to resolvins in the body. These compounds are 10,000 times more effective than normal fatty acids. They inhibit the functioning of immune system mediators that cause inflammation.

For inflammation to occur, the body has its own on and off switch. Omega 3s inhibit the turning on of these switches so that the inflammatory pathway cannot proceed.

Hyaluronic Acid

Hyaluronic acid is a component of synovial fluid which is present between joints and allows easy gliding of bones. In patients of rheumatoid arthritis, this component starts to break up and functioning of the fluid is affected.

While its primary administration is through injections as a pain reliever, the same is also found in small doses in supplements. Research shows that low dioses of this acid can reduce chronic pain and joint stiffness, though results may vary from person to person.

You can take hyaluronic acid for knee osteoarthritis in the form of 50mg tablets twice a day with meals. If your case is more severe, your doctor may recommend an injection.

It incorporates into the synovial fluid and reduces friction between the bones, causing them to brush against each other swiftly. In this way, it reduces stiffness of joints and enhances mobility.

Hyaluronic acid is especially used for the treatment of knee, hip and ankle arthritis as these are the regions where joints are extremely critical. The ball and socket joint in the hips that provide maximum mobility can often be affected due to arthritis. So this supplement helps rebuild the shock-absorbing fluid present in the joints and acts like grease in bones.

Hyaluronic acid injections are prescribed for patients when pain from knee arthritis can no longer be controlled by anti-inflammatory drugs and NSAIDS.

CHAPTER 8

OTHER JOINT PAIN TREATMENT OPTIONS

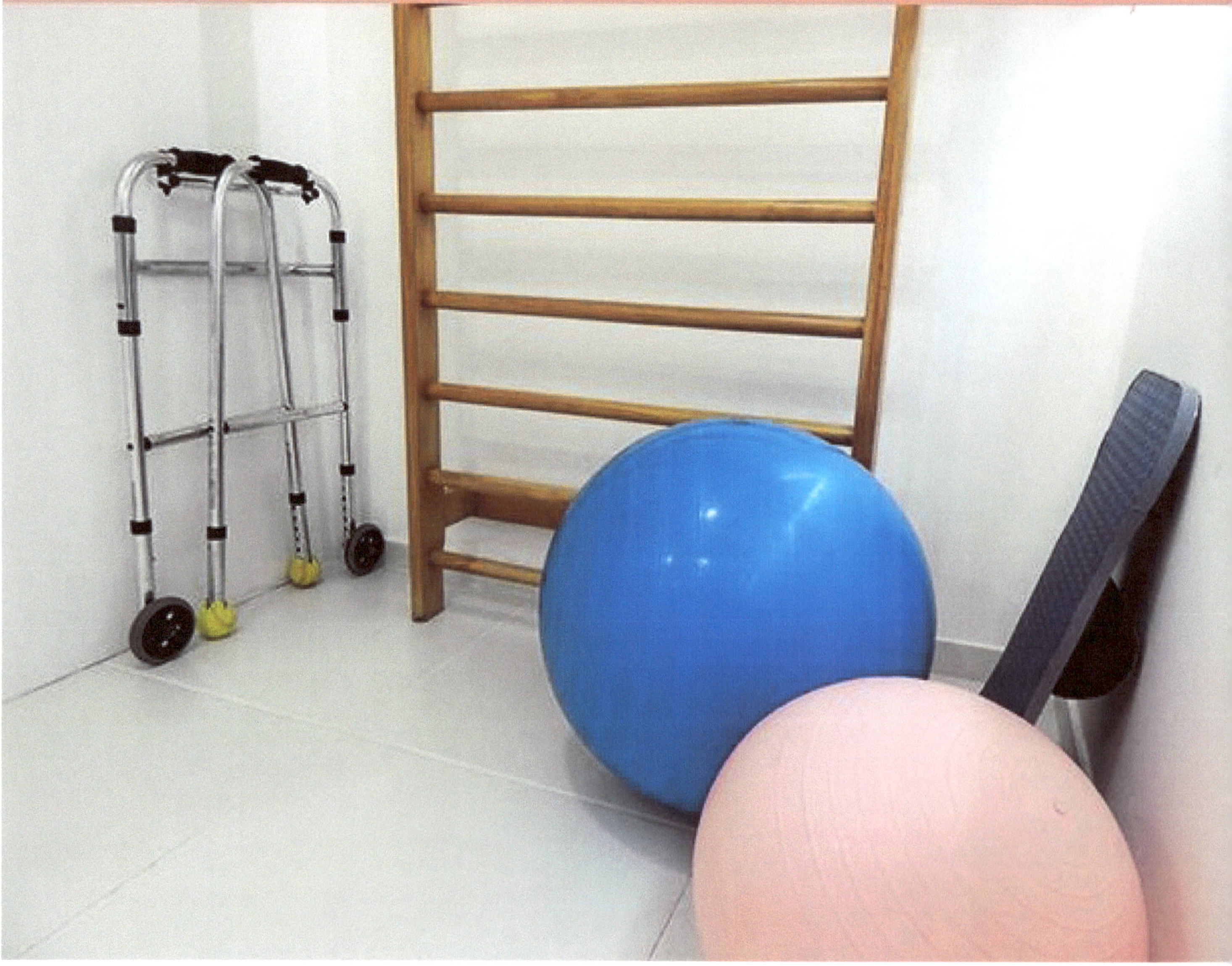

Chapter 8

Other Joint Pain Treatment Options

When your joint pain becomes bothersome to a greater extent, you can get help from some other options including the following:

Medications as a Last Resort

Analgesics or painkillers are the most common medications used for joint pain. Tylenol is a common drug which contains Acetaminophen. According to many guidelines, this drug is the first line of defense against knee or hip pain associated with osteoarthritis. However, you may experience some side effects after extended use of Tylenol.

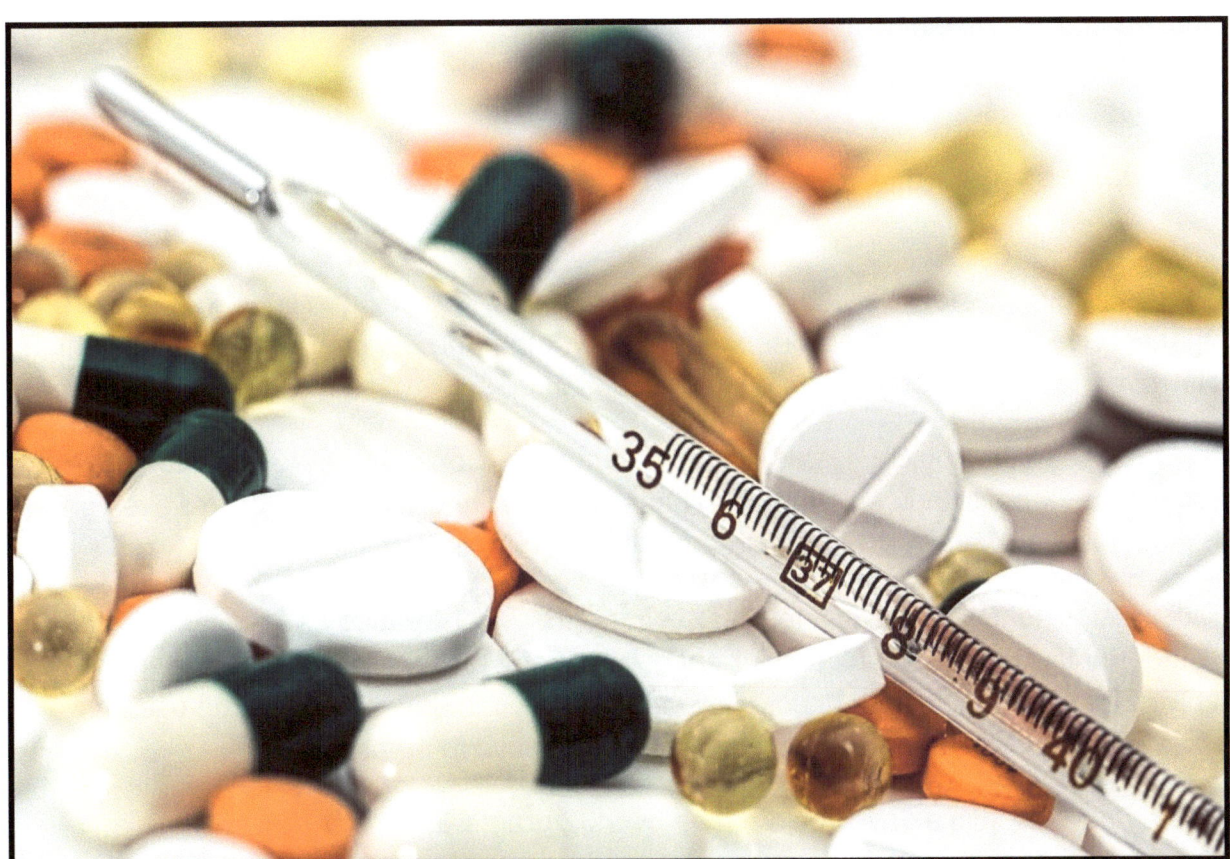

Side effects of this drug include gastrointestinal bleedings, ulcers and loss of kidney functions. It is recommended to lower the dosage or lessen the treatment time.

For people who are already suffering from diseases such as blood pressure, diabetes or cardiovascular diseases, the amount of Acetaminophen advised for them is uncertain. This doesn't mean that they can't use the drug for treatment; it just means that they need to consult their doctors to set a dosage.

NSAIDS or Non-Steroid Anti-inflammatory drugs are also used for pain relief in arthritis. Some examples of these drugs include aspirin and ibuprofen. The problem, however, is that the likelihood of side effects is higher with NSAIDS as compared to acetaminophen. NSAIDs can also cause kidney damage and can harm the cardiovascular system.

Diacerein is a slow-acting drug for reducing the damage to cartilage. This drug is prescribed to people with osteoarthritis. Although the drug is more effective than placebo, it increases the risk of diarrhea.

Duloxetine is an anti-depressant that is given to osteoarthritis patients. It's thought to help with chronic joint pain. It also has side effects such as dry mouth, fatigue, sweating, nausea and constipation.

Topical Agents

Topical treatments for relieving joint pain include gels, patches and liquid. Topical agents have different strengths depending on whether the pain is low, moderate or high. However, these are not given without prescription.

It's been seen that topical agents have the same effect on pain as NSAIDs but they have more benefits than side effects. These agents might not be suitable for everyone but people who want to avoid oral treatments can benefit from them.

Diclofenac sodium 1% gel is a topical gel that is used for treating patients of osteoarthritis. This gel is suitable for hand, wrists and elbow arthritis. The patient has to apply 2 grams of the gel on affected area four times in a day. It can also be used for knee or ankle arthritis but then 4 grams of the gel have to be applied.

The amount used in a day should not be over 32 grams. When you buy the gel, a dosing card accompanies it so you can measure the amount for daily usage.

A diclofenac epolamine 1.3% patch is also available for pain relief. You just have to apply the patch twice a day to the painful joint. Topical treatments may also be in form of drops such as diclofenac sodium 2% liquid. To apply this, you have to put 40 drops on each knee four times in a day, as it is best for knee arthritis.

Other than these topical treatments, NSAIDs such as ibuprofen can also be made into topical solutions. Topical agents are best for joints that are closer to the surface. So, they'll help relieve pain that comes with hand, elbows and ankle arthritis.

Those who can't take oral medication because they are diabetic or have heart problems can use topical agents instead. Likewise, people who have a history of gastrointestinal problems or ulcers should opt for topical agents rather than oral NSAIDs.

Injections

Injections are the middle ground between surgery and oral medication. If oral NSAIDs don't work for you and you're not yet ready for surgery, then injections are your fix. Hyaluronic acid injections are given for knee arthritis to supplement the natural hyaluronic acid present in the joints.

When injected into a joint, it helps reduce pain and inflammation. These injections are given three to five times a week. The doctor would first insert an empty syringe into the knee to remove fluid from the knee to make room for hyaluronic acid. Then, hyaluronic acid supplement is injected into the emptied area.

Corticosteroid injections are also given for reducing pain and inflammation. These injections are also given directly and are most suitable for knee osteoarthritis. The benefit of these injections can last for a few weeks or even six months.

Although these injections don't have as many side effects as oral medications, it doesn't mean that they have no risks associated with them. Doctors normally limit the number of injections you get since excessive use of these injections can actually contribute to cartilage breakdown.

Arthrocentesis is a process in which a hollow needle is inserted into the joint and the joint fluid is removed. Oftentimes, this fluid is removed so that it can be tested in labs but when excess fluid is removed, pain and inflammation is also sufficiently reduced. Sometimes, doctors can insert corticosteroid injections into the same place from where the joint fluid was removed.

Physical Therapy

Physical therapy is a great tool for reducing stiffness that comes with joint pain. Occupational therapists can train patients to move their affected joints without increasing any pain. Also, they help patients change their homes to adapt to their needs.

With physical therapy, stress on joints is reduced. Sometimes, splints or other devices are also suggested to help the patient in daily tasks like dressing and driving.

The aim of physical therapy is to ensure that you can perform daily chores without any difficulty. Your therapist would try to increase the range of motion and build strength in the areas around joints. This increases flexibility and motion.

A physical therapist teaches you how to do simple chores in a way that least stress is put on joints and stiffness is reduced. Since every patient is different, a therapist would devise a personalized exercise plan for you. It'll teach you how to maintain proper posture and use assistive devices such as canes or splints.

A physical therapist would also tell you how to properly use a heat or cold treatment method and bring some ergonomic changes to your house. For example, a therapist might suggest you use cushioned mats or get special chairs.

After frequent visits to a physical therapist, you'll be able to do things like reach your kitchen cabinets, bend down to tie your shoelace and take a morning walk.

Over time, if you consistently do the exercises, your body will get adept at the routine and get stronger. You can get recommendations from your doctor about a therapist or you can find one in your area who specializes in arthritis patients.

Remember that you must combine the treatment methods to get the best results, rather than just relying on any single one.

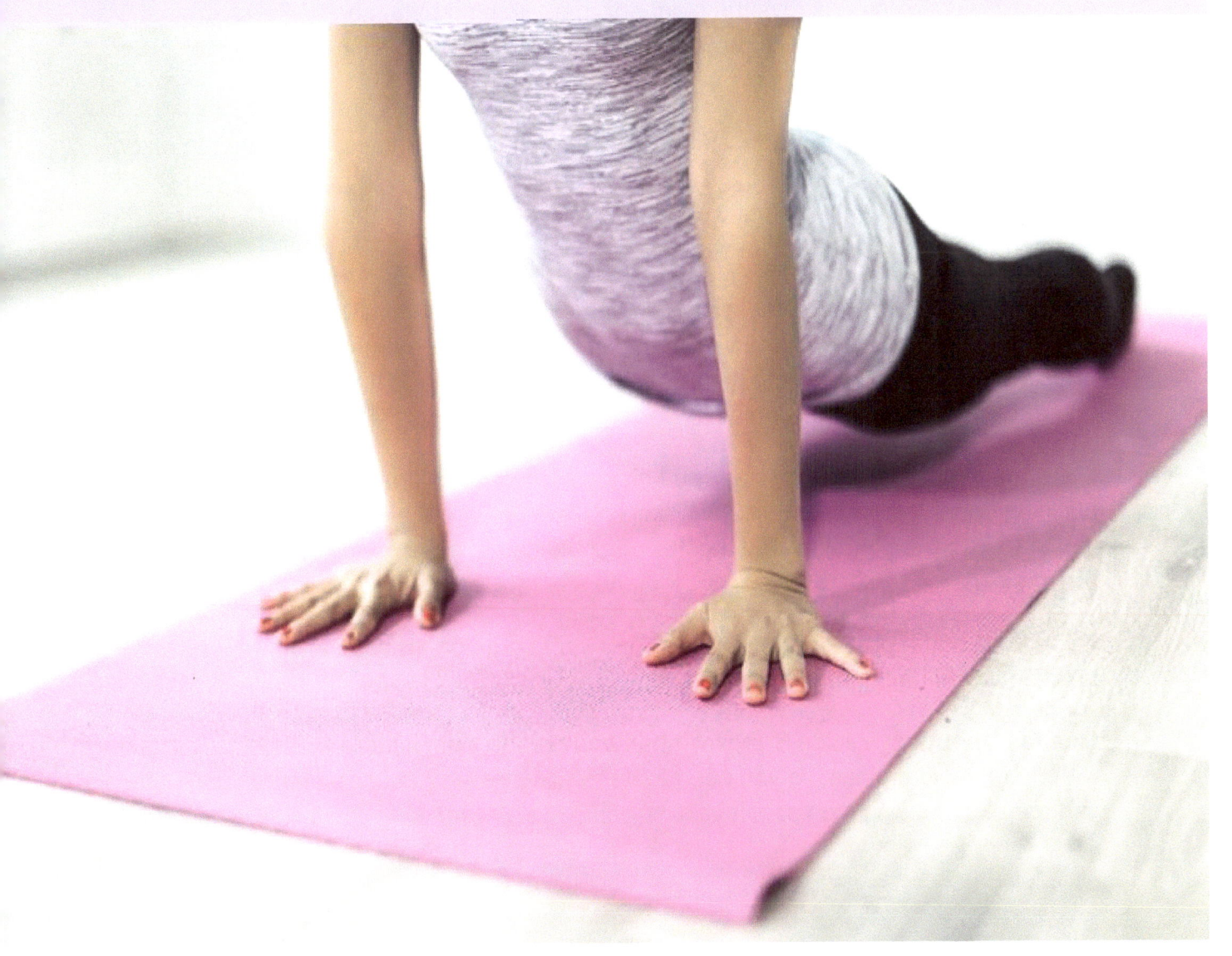

Conclusion

CONCLUSION
TO
JOINT HEALTH

Conclusion

When you have arthritis of any kind, your life can be a physical and emotional rollercoaster. You have more bad days than good days and it's hard just to go on. You remember that you used to do so much and now you need to have other people help you just to do the basic chores around the house. The damage to your joints keeps degenerating more all the time and limits you with pain and stiffness. You want a way out.

One of the first things to do is to keep moving. Your joints will benefit from the movement and that will keep them lubricated and flexible as much as possible. You will get some freedom back but it will be slow going. You must keep your spirits up. Do what you can but keep walking and bending.

Second, you must keep your nutrition high. Labeled as a "cooked food disease", arthritics need to forgo the empty calories and eat food that is as fresh and close to raw as possible. Cooking destroys the plant enzymes needed by the body. Fresh greens will be the basis of your meal with protein and other vegetables to fill in. A nutritional approach will help alleviate most of the symptoms and pain.

Next, you must keep hydrated. Your joints need fluid and after you hydrate the rest of your body then you need to drink extra for your joints. Water is the first thing you should drink everyday. Drink the purest water you can. You can buy water filters for your home and carry it in water bottles with you.

Stop Smoking! Smoking releases toxins and excess free radicals into the body. These attack the immune system and white blood cells. Over a long time, the bones are affected by the toxins and lose the ability to repair the damage; this can lead to a breakdown of bone in the joints.

Lose the excess weight. You are putting too much weight on your joints and they are buckling under the pressure. Not only will you feel better but also your pain will stop if you start losing weight now. Putting this off could cause damage in your joints that is irreversible.

If you have had a **previous joint injury**, it is very common for osteoarthritis to develop in the joint you had damaged.

One last thought: Suicide is prevalent among chronic pain sufferers, especially those with rheumatoid arthritis, so you need to be aware of your thought patterns during times you are experiencing high pain levels.

Promise yourself that you will not do anything for 24 hours if your thoughts are turning to suicide. If you need to talk to someone about how you feel and the pain you are experiencing reach out online, by telephone to a family member or a friend, or to a hotline for help. Even your doctor may have a way to help you. Just don't go it alone. Try the recommendations above and build a support group around you for help.

While exercise and diet remain the fundamentals for good joint health, you can also include things like supplements and physical or aquatic therapy to enhance your joint health.

Preventing joint pain can be a lot easier than having to deal with the distress of joint inflammation and susceptibility to disease. Let your joints thank you for taking good care of them!

About the Author

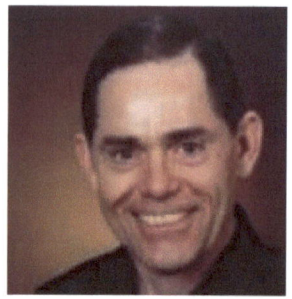

I have published numerous books on Amazon (both for Kindle and in paperback), along with other publishing platforms.

While most of my books are on health and fitness in general, I also write on baby boomer and older citizen health issues and have a recent interest in creating and printing journals/ planners and other printable products. A complete list of our published products on Amazon can be found at https://www.amazon.com/Ron-Kness/e/B0072M6PYO.

Besides my own writing, I also ghostwrite ebooks, books, reports, articles, blogs and do Kindle conversions for clients on a variety of topics. Contact me at Ron Kness Writing for a quote.

Today my wife and I are retired from our careers and live in Gold Canyon, AZ. I now write as a retirement business where you'll find me happily sitting in my office typing away on my laptop as I work on my next book or ghostwriting project . . . that is if we are not traveling on a cruise ship - our new-found mode of travel.